Clinical Cases for
MRCPCH Foundation in Practice

July 2017

RCPCH

Royal College of
Paediatrics and Child Health

Leading the way in Children's Health

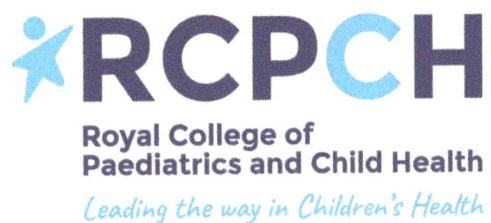

Foreword

This new textbook from the UK Royal College of Paediatrics and Child Health contains 50 chapters covering the Foundation of Practice syllabus. Each chapter contains questions similar to those used in the exam, with answers, discussion, references and suggestions for further reading.

The Foundation of Practice examination is taken by MRCPCH and DCH candidates in the UK and abroad. The authors include both established consultants as well as paediatricians in training, so you can be assured that the content reflects contemporaneous paediatric practice.

I found the book enjoyable and stimulating and was struck as much by the readability of the style as the day-to-day relevance of the content; this is no compendium of esoteric medical rarities, but a practical aid to everyday paediatrics. The authors and editors are to be congratulated for producing an excellent resource. This textbook will stand you in good stead for the MRCPCH examinations, but above all, I believe you will find it an enjoyable and stimulating read.

Professor Neena Modi

President Royal College of Paediatrics and Child Health

Preface

The aim of the Foundation of Practice examination is to assess your knowledge, understanding and clinical decision making abilities for commonly presenting paediatric problems. The exam is the first step towards achieving either the Diploma in Child Health or your Membership of the Royal College of Paediatrics and Child Health.

I have been involved with the membership examinations for the past 12 years, and vice chair for the Foundation of Practice examination for the past 4 years. When I first became involved in the exam boards, it struck me that some of the questions were not so relevant to my experience as a trainee doctor. I had never seen Renal Tubular Acidosis Type 4 or Niemann-Pick disease, yet I was expecting trainee doctors with 6 months of paediatric experience to be able to answer questions about them in a high pressure exam. The exam always had a question about Kawasaki's (which I had seen once or twice) but rarely questions about bronchiolitis, or eczema, or parents concerned about their newborn baby crying, or drunk teenagers, which is what I saw in my day-to-day job as a junior doctor. In the last decade or so the biggest improvement in the postgraduate exams, in my view, is that the questions have become more "real", reflecting the experiences we have as doctors.

The boundless knowledge contained within the World Wide Web means that medical information is available within a few clicks. Every doctor now uses the information contained to gain knowledge of rare conditions which one encounters. It would be churlish to ask you about the clinical feature of GM1 gangliosidoses in your membership exams when in clinical practise you would wisely use the internet to review this condition. However, it would be reasonable to expect that you had a good grasp of the management of acute emergencies or commonly presenting paediatric conditions. Furthermore, whilst the web can give you information it can't tell you how to apply that knowledge in specific circumstances. It is with this in mind that the questions used in both the theory examinations and this book is written.

The purpose of this book is to provide you with a series of clinically based questions identical in format to those which are used in the current computer based exam. The questions give as broad a view as possible of the type of clinical scenarios which are likely to be encountered in the exam and all syllabus areas have been covered.

Each chapter is based on a typical clinical scenario followed by questions relevant to the topic. A succinct review of the subject is then given interspersed with carefully chosen references relevant to the topic under discussion which should also act as suggestions for further reading. The chapters have been written by paediatricians, both consultants and those in training, and all chapters have been reviewed by individuals involved in the theory examinations. You can be certain therefore that the questions in this book are of a similar standard and format to those used in the actual exam.

The best way to use this book is not to read it from cover to cover all at once. Each chapter should be reviewed individually by reading the case history, attempting the questions and learning from the accompanying discussion of the relevant subject. This can be done individually or in group sessions with other colleagues.

A huge thank you is due to all of the authors for their time in writing the chapters, their enthusiasm, patience and hard work sharing their huge personal experience and knowledge. In addition, this book would not have been possible without the excellent team at the RCPCH Quality and Standards team, especially Sheran Mahal who kept me on track and saved the book from my organisational inabilities on several occasions.

Finally, I want to thank you for either undertaking a career in paediatrics and/or taking an interest in the health needs of children. In the modern world there has never been a greater need for advocates for children and I encourage you to learn, help, laugh and play with as many of them as possible!

Dr Chris Dewhurst

Vice Chair Foundation of Practice MRCPCH Examination

Contents

Chapter 1: Day 1 in the children's emergency department
Dr Simon Li

It is your first shift in the emergency department and the following children are brought into the department:

This is a list of ingestions:

A.	Antifreeze	F.	Digoxin
B.	Aspirin	G.	Iron tablets
C.	Bleach	H.	Metal coin
D.	Button battery	I.	Morphine
E.	Diazepam	J.	Paracetamol

For each of the following clinical scenarios choose the most likely ingestion:

Q1a. A 16 year old girl is vomiting and complaining of abdominal pain. After the results of her blood tests come back she commences N-acetylcysteine.

Q1b. An 18 month old boy is vomiting after being found in the kitchen with an open bottle and the liquid it contained spread over the floor. He has some oral ulceration but he is otherwise happily playing in the waiting area. He is encouraged to drink milk.

Q1c. A 2 year girl says that "her tummy hurts". Whilst she is in the emergency department she has several episodes of vomiting with subsequent haematemesis. On assessment she looks pale and clammy, with a heart rate of 154/minute and a blood pressure of 102/56 mmHg. A metal detector passed over her chest is positive above the diaphragm.

A 2 year old girl is brought into the emergency department. Her mum states that she was playing in the kitchen when she reached out to a pan containing boiling water that was resting on the hob which tipped over her.

Q2. What is the next best step in her management?

A.	Apply a bag of ice and water on the affected arm
B.	Apply a cold wet flannel on the affected arm
C.	Direct an electric fan on to the affected arm
D.	Place the girl into a bath of cool water
E.	Run cool tap water over the affected arm for 20 minutes

Q3. Which one of the following would make you suspicious of a non-accidental burn?

A.	It affects both her hands and feet circumferentially
B.	It has an irregular shaped margin to it
C.	It predominantly affects the front of her body
D.	It shows asymmetric involvement
E.	It varies in superficial, partial and full thickness burn depth

Answers and Rationale

Q1a. J: Paracetamol
Q1b. C: Bleach
Q1c. D: Button battery
Q2. E: Run cool tap water over the affected arm for 20 minutes
Q3. A: It affects both her hands and feet circumferentially

Although England has one of the highest child mortality rates in Europe for those aged between 0-14 years of old, it has the fifth lowest mortality rate as a result of accidents. Road traffic accidents constitute over one-third of these accidental deaths of which 50% are cyclists (1). Other common causes of accidental death are shown in (table 1.1). This extended matching question focuses on poisonings which, in the context of accidents, accounts for 8% of deaths.

The first question focuses on a teenager who presents with rather non-specific symptoms of vomiting and abdominal pain which may relate to any number of ingestions from the list. The answer lies in knowing the management of the most common poisonings, in this case knowing that acetylcysteine treats paracetamol overdose.

The second part of this question describes a rather common scenario of young, mobile children. The advent of child safety locks on the cupboard has reduced this situation but not completely. The examination of the child is unremarkable save for oral ulceration. Moreover milk has been advised to counteract the ingestion. It is most likely that he has drunk bleach. Incidentally the milk works by being digested by the stomach acids which causes it to curdle within the stomach. This curdled milk coats the stomach and slows down the rate with which the bleach is absorbed.

The third question describes a girl with abdominal pain and vomiting which again are rather non-specific features that do not really help in the diagnosis. What is worrying however is the haematemesis she has developed which has led to her haemodynamic instability. The give-away here is a positive test with the metal detector. Out of the list given this really can only be a button battery. The public are rather naïve when it comes to these objects as they are deemed innocuous perhaps because of their small size. However their danger results when they get stuck within the oesophagus or do not move when they enter the bowel because of the high risk of mucosal erosion when the battery acid is released from the battery casing.

The other ingestions from the list vary in their management. Initially all children should be assessed and managed according to APLS guidelines so as to identify whether the child is symptomatic of the potentially poisoned child. Specific management is divided into general supportive therapy and more specific therapy in whom it is indicated. A number of antidotes are available to aid in the management some of which are shown in (Table 1.2) (2).

Burns and scalds to children are common with 70% of accidental childhood burns and scalds occurring in those under 3 years of age. All burns should initially be managed according to ATLS protocols with the thorough and timely assessment of the airway, breathing and circulation.

Once this has occurred the priority should then be to remove the patient from the source of the burn, including the removal of any clothing unless it is adherent to the patient. Following this the affected area should be cooled by running cool water over it for 20 minutes. This gold standard of first aid reduces the severity of tissue damage as well as relieving associated pain as it is not exposed to air. Durations of cooling greater than 30 minutes have not been shown to be beneficial and although it is best to immerse the affected area immediately, there appears to be benefit even with a delay of up to 3 hours. Following this a temporary dressing, such as cling film, should be applied before getting further medical assessment. Larger wounds should be covered with a wet dressing as immersion of a child in cold water to avert wound injury progression is outweighed by the risks of hypothermia (3).

Once the child has been stabilised and initial treatment provided thoughts must turn, as always in paediatrics, as to whether concerns about safeguarding and a child's wellbeing should be raised. Although each injury should be judged on an individual basis there are certain patterns of injury that are more consistent with accidental scalds. These are those burns that have an irregular margin and burn depth and when there is asymmetric involvement. The mechanism of injury must also fit with the pattern of the burn. In Q3 you are not told where the burn has affected her but given that she has reached out to the pan of water, a burn that affects the front of her body would be more in keeping with this story than a burn which affected her posteriorly. Here the answer must be a burn that affects her hands and feet which is not in keeping with the mechanism of injury. Indeed burns that only affect the hands and feet circumferentially in the glove and stocking distribution are highly characteristic of intentional scalds (4).

Incident type	<1	1-4	5-9	10-14	Total
			Age		
Road transport	1	25	21	44	91
Drowning/choking/suffocation	1	11	1	4	17
Fire	0	6	2	2	10
Poisoning	0	2	1	5	8
Falls	0	2	1	5	8
Other	25	18	10	20	73

Table 1.1: Overview of unintentional injury deaths by age and mechanism, England and Wales 2008

Poisoning agent	Presentation	Antidote	Mechanism of action
Antifreeze (ethylene glycol)	Cranial nerve palsies, renal impairment, metabolic acidosis	Fomepizole, ethanol	Competitive inhibitor of alcohol dehydrogenase preventing toxic metabolite production
Digoxin	Bradycardia with ECG changes, blurred vision, xanthopsia	Digoxin specific antibody fragments	Binds digoxin preventing interaction with target sites
Benzodiazepines	Ataxia, blurred vision, sedation, hallucinations, slurred speech, nysatgmus	Flumazenil	Benzodiazepine receptor site antagonist
Iron	Gastrointestinal haemorrhage	Desferrioxamine	Binds free iron and enhances renal elimination
Opioids e.g. morphine	Hypoventilation, hypotension, mioisism sedation, bradycardia	Naloxone	Competitive antagonist at the opioid receptor

Table 1.2: Examples of presentation and antidotes

Syllabus Mapping

Emergency Medicine (including accidents and poisoning)

- Know about immediate care for children with burns and scalds, recognising that they may be a presentation of non-accidental injury

- Be aware of common causes of accidents in children and adolescents including safeguarding implications and understand prevention strategies

- Know the common causes of poisoning in children and adolescents including safeguarding implications

Pharmacology

- Know how to prescribe safely and be aware of adverse effects and interactions of drugs

Safeguarding

- Know the presentations of physical, emotional and sexual abuse, neglect and fabricated and induced illness

References and Further Reading

1. Patel D, Sandell JM. Prevention of unintentional injury in children. Paediatrics and Child Health 2013;23(9):402-08

2. Anderson M. The management of poisoning. Paediatrics and Child Health 2013;23(9):380-84

3. Goutos I, Tyler M. Early management of paediatric burn injuries. Paediatrics and Child Health 2013;23(9):391-96

4. Maguire S, Okolie C, Kemp AM. Burns as a consequence of child maltreatment. Paediatrics and Child Health 2014;24(12):557-61

Chapter 2: A child with a limp and a swollen joint
Dr Beverley Almeida

You are reviewing patients in the rapid access clinic. Your next patient is Lara, a 4 year old girl with a 6 week history of right hip pain that wakes her up at night. Lara was diagnosed with developmental dysplasia of the hip (DDH) at 14 months after she started walking. This was surgically treated.

Q1. Which one of the following findings on clinical examination in a 14 month old would best support a diagnosis of DDH?

A. Affected leg appears longer than the other
B. Affected leg appears shorter than the other
C. Bottom shuffling
D. Walking on their tip toes
E. Walking with an antalgic gait

Her mother had initially attributed the recent hip pain to "growing pains" and the previously treated DDH. Since waiting for the appointment Lara has developed a swollen right knee. On further questioning, you discover that she has been bruising easily and has had quite a few viral illnesses in the last few months.

On examination she walks with a right sided limp and has an antalgic gait. She has a swollen right knee which is tender and has slightly restricted movement. On standing there is evidence of genu valgus. A full joint examination reveals no other affected joints. She has many bruises and a few petechiae on her ankles. There are no other rashes. She has pale conjunctiva.

You arrange the following blood tests: full blood count (FBC) and urea and electrolytes (U&Es), the results of which are pending.

Q2. Which one of the following is the most important next investigation?

A. Anti-nuclear antibodies (ANA)
B. Arthrocentesis with fluid microscopy and culture
C. Blood film
D. C-reactive protein (CRP)
E. Erythrocyte sedimentation rate (ESR)

Q3. What is the most likely diagnosis?

A. Acute lymphoblastic leukaemia (ALL)
B. Henoch-Schönlein purpura (HSP)
C. Juvenile idiopathic arthritis (JIA)
D. Non-accidental injury
E. Reactive arthritis

Answers and Rationale

Q1.   B: Affected leg appears shorter than the other
Q2.   C: Blood film
Q3.   A: Acute lymphoblastic leukaemia (ALL)

In this case, developmental dysplasia of the hip (DDH) is a coincidental finding. DDH occurs due to disruption of the normal relationship between the femoral head and the acetabulum. DDH is more common in girls and first born babies. Risk factors include a positive family history, prematurity, multiple birth, breech position during the last stages of pregnancy, oligohydraminos and neuromuscular disease. All babies are screened for DDH at the routine newborn and 6 week examinations. A positive test is indicated if the hip is able to be dislocated (Barlow test, the hip is able to be "popped out") and/or a dislocated hip is able to be put back into joint (Otolani test, when a "clunk" is felt as a dislocated hip slips back into joint). Asymmetry of the skin creases and limb length discrepancies may also be present. A positive screening test and/or the presence of risk factors warrant a hip ultrasound scan (USS). If the USS is normal then baby can be discharged, if the USS is abnormal referral to orthopaedic surgeons is required.

DDH may not be detected in the newborn period but present later. Sometimes DDH may remain undetected through until adulthood. Signs in an older child include restricted movement in one leg during nappy changes, the leg dragging behind the other when crawling, the affected leg appearing shorter than the other, uneven skin folds in the buttocks or thighs, limping, tip-toe walking or an abnormal gait. Hip USSs are not able to detect DDH once the proximal femoral epiphysis has ossified (approximately 6 months) and therefore plain x-ray is the investigation of choice in the older infant and child.

DDH is usually treated with an abduction brace if detected early and by surgery (either open or closed reduction or acetabuloplasty) if detected late. The outcome and prognosis are good if the diagnosis is made early and the treatment is prompt. The later the DDH is detected the worse the outcome. If not detected or detected in late childhood limb-length discrepancy with a flexion/adduction deformity of the hip, postural scoliosis, back pain and ipsilateral genu valgum with consequent arthritis of the knee may occur.

When Lara returns at 4 years old with pallor, bruising, petechiae and recurrent infections, you should have a high index of suspicion for leukaemia. Bone pain, myalgia and joint symptoms are also relatively common presentations of malignancy, leukaemia in particular. A full blood count (FBC) will show pancytopaenia with a decrease in the counts for all three cell lines – red blood cells, white blood cells and platelets. A blood film will demonstrate lymphoblast which is helpful in the initial diagnosis, although referral to a tertiary oncology centre for a diagnostic bone marrow aspirate and trephine should be made. Oral or intravenous steroids should definitely be avoided until these investigations have been completed and certainly should only be administered under the supervision of a Paediatric Oncologist. The associated arthritis in malignancy usually resolves quickly with the initiation of appropriate chemotherapeutic treatment.

Juvenile idiopathic arthritis (JIA) is the most common chronic rheumatologic disease in children. The aetiology is unknown and there are several different subtypes including systemic-onset, oligoarticular and polyarticular. For JIA to be diagnosed the arthritis must be present for > 6 weeks. A diagnosis of reactive arthritis (arthritis following viral illnesses) is more common prior to this 6 week cut-off.

The bruising of different ages should always make you think of non-accidental injury (NAI), however in view of the pallor and recurrent infections, does not fit. Swollen joints can be seen in NAI due to trauma and limps due to fractures. The symptoms of bruising in conjunction with a swollen joint could also raise the possibility of haemophilia, but this is X-linked recessive and is almost exclusively seen in boys. Henoch-Schönlein purpura (HSP) can often cause arthritis but is associated with palpable purpura and not petechiae or bruising. However, in the case of an isolated single swollen joint associated with fever (i.e. absence of bruising and recurrent viral illness) an infective cause should be ruled out first, most commonly staphylococcus, and streptococcus so an anti-streptolysin titre (ASOT) is helpful.

Assessment, causes and initial management of joint swelling

If swollen joints persist for longer than 6 weeks, the diagnosis of JIA should be considered and a referral to a Paediatric Rheumatologist should be made. A full musculoskeletal history and examination of the joints, tendons and muscles will be carried out. Inflammatory markers such as the c-reactive protein (CRP) and erythrocyte sedimentation rate (ESR) are helpful as an indication of the level of inflammation, but if they are grossly raised then infection should be suspected. Simple x-rays or ultrasound of the affected joints are helpful in aiding the diagnosis (the hip, sacroiliac and back and temperomandibular joints tend to be better imaged with magnetic resonance imaging (MRI)). An anti-nuclear antibody (ANA) gives an indication if the patient is more at risk of developing uveitis, although all patients with JIA are routinely reviewed by ophthalmology. A rheumatoid factor does not help make the diagnosis but if positive gives an indication that the patient may have a more prolonged disease course and poorer prognosis.

Some types of JIA are associated with skin manifestations, such as systemic JIA, but this is commonly a salmon pink rash that comes and goes with spikes of fever rather than bruising or petechiae. Psoriatic JIA can be seen with nail changes or typical plaques or a family history of a 1st degree relative with psoriasis.

Differential diagnosis of pain on walking and limp

In Lara's case the pain in the right hip is most likely referred pain from the right knee. Referred pain which is very common in younger children who find it difficult to localize pain, however pain that wakes the child during the night is a red flag and may actually represent bony pain. An antalgic gait means there is pain on walking as the child minimizes weight bearing on the sore limb. Most limps occur due to a new condition (Table 2.1), but if a child has always had a limp since starting to walk consider an undiagnosed developmental dysplasia of the hip (DDH) or neurological conditions such as cerebral palsy (CP).

Cause	Conditions
Trauma	Toddler's fracture, non-accidental injury
Infection	Osteomyelitis, septic arthritis
Malignancy	Neuroblastoma, acute lymphoblasticlLeukaemia, bone tumours
Surgical	Testicular torsion, inguinal hernia, appendicitis,
Structural	Osgood-Schlatter disease, Perthes disease, slipped upper femoral epiphysis (SUFE), DDH
Inflammatory	JIA, transient synovitis, reactive arthritis, lyme arthritis
Metabolic	Rickets
Neurological	CP
Haematological	Sickle cell anaemia

Table 2.1: Causes and conditions presenting with a limp

Normal variations of limb development

Lara also has genu valgum (knock knees). This has occurred due to the pathology of the swollen right knee joint. However, genu valgum, genu varus, in-toeing and flat feet are normal variations of limb development up to certain ages as set out in (Table 2.2).

Variation	Description	Normal in children	Associated with	Treatment
Genu valgum (knock knees)	Large gap between feet when standing with knees together	Up to the age of 6	Rickets Obesity Late feature of arthritis of the knee	May need referral to orthopaedics if the intermalleolar distance is >6cm or persists >6 years
Genu varus (bow legs)	Bowing of the lower leg in relation to the thigh	Up to the age of 2	Rickets Skeletal dysplasias Achrondoplasia Dwarfism Late feature of arthritis of the knee	May need referral to orthopaedics if the intercondylar distance is >6cm or persists >6 years
In-toeing	Toes point inward when walking, due to the feet, femur or tibia	Femoral anterversion usually correct by age 14. Tibial torsion usually corrects by age 5	None	If in-toeing is due to the feet, metatarsus adductus and the foot is not flexible then plaster casts or minor surgery may be used to correct the problem.
Mobile flat feet	Absence of arch on standing flat, becomes apparent when on tiptoes	Up to the age of 8	Hypermobility	Reassurance and footwear advice. Occasionally insoles or physiotherapy
Joint hypermobility	Great range of joint mobility to that which is usually expected. Usually asymptomatic, although some individuals experience pain	Up to the age of 5	Mobile flat feet Tight hamstrings	Can be used to the individual's advantage e.g. ballet or gymnastics. Reassurance. May require physiotherapy and muscle strengthening exercises, occupational therapy and psychology support.

Table 2.2: Normal musculoskeletal Variants

Syllabus Mapping

Musculoskeletal

- Know the normal variations of limb development e.g. bow legs and knock knees, in-toeing, flat feet

- Know about the assessment, causes and initial management of joint and limb pain, joint laxity and swelling

- Know the differential diagnosis of pain on walking and limp and initial management

- Know the causes of acute and chronic arthritis including those with systemic manifestations (e.g. Henoch-Schönlein purpura) and understand the principles of management

- Know how to recognise developmental dysplasia of the hip, appropriate referral pathways and usual management

Haematology and Oncology

- Know the clinical manifestations of acute leukaemia, lymphoma, and solid tumours

References and Further Reading

1. Foster HE, Brogan PA. Paediatric rheumatology. Oxford University Press; 2012 Jun 14

2. Smith E, Anderson M, Foster H. The child with a limp: a symptom and not a diagnosis. Archives of disease in childhood: Education & practice edition. 2012 Jul 21

Chapter 3: A busy day on the ward
Dr Michelle Arora, Dr Natalie Bee and Dr Julie-Clare Becher

3

You are working on the general paediatric ward and are about to perform a lumbar puncture under aseptic conditions on Sai, a 6 month old baby girl, when you are bleeped. You ask one of the support workers to answer it while you and the nurse continue with the procedure. The support worker returns to tell you that the microbiology lab have called to say that the nasopharyngeal secretions taken from a 3 month old boy in bay 4 are positive for pertussis. On admission, Sai was respiratory syncytial virus (RSV) positive on near-patient testing. He is currently being nursed in the RSV cohort bay and you were not aware pertussis testing had been requested. You are still undertaking the lumbar puncture so you are unable to act on this information at present. You tell the support worker you will address this after completing the procedure. You complete the lumbar puncture, document the procedure in the notes and update Sai's parents. You are thereafter bleeped repeatedly with multiple GP referrals and you forget about his result. You are not on shift the next day. The day team chase the nasopharyngeal aspirate result and find that Sai is positive for pertussis. They identify that this requires the patient to be isolated and commenced on treatment. The microbiology department have informed public health department.

Q1. What should be the team's next most important management step?

A.   Complete a clinical incident form
B.   Inform Infection Control and Occupational Health
C.   Inform the referring unit (the emergency department)
D.   Prescribe clarithromycin for clinical staff
E.   Prescribe clarithromycin for other patients in the bay

Q2. Which human factors was the root cause of this error?

A.   Inability to prioritise
B.   Ineffective communication
C.   Ineffective time management
D.   Mismanagement of a heavy workload
E.   Poor situation awareness

Q3. Which of the following is the best improvement that can be made to avoid such events in the future?

A.   Ensure all staff on the ward complete a communication course
B.   Ensure that results of Public Health importance are communicated to more senior clinical staff
C.   Establish a rule that procedures are made distraction-free
D.   None. It was a one-off human error which could not happen again
E.   Prevent clinical support workers from answering clinicians bleeps

Answers and Rationale

Q1.   **E: Prescribe clarithromycin for other patients in the bay**
Q2.   **B: Ineffective communication**
Q3.   **C: Establish a rule that procedures are made distraction-free**

The Foundation of Practice examination not only includes clinical questions but also those involving professional and governance issues. In all scenarios, the health and safety of patients under your care is your immediate priority. All the answers to question 1 are management plans that should be implemented in this scenario however the immediate patient safety issue is to protect your patients. Young infants, especially babies less than 3 months old, and partially immunised infants (less than 12 months old) are at the greatest risk of severe complications of pertussis infection (1). Current recommendations are that all non-immunised and partially immunised children (<12 months old) admitted to the same bay need to be offered clarithromycin as prophylaxis. Some contacts may also be eligible for post-exposure vaccination (2).

Some hospital laboratories would routinely inform the Infection Prevention and Control Team (IPCT) in this scenario. However, you need to ensure this has been done. The IPCT and Occupational Health (OH) need to consider prophylaxis for other patients and staff who have been exposed (2). This includes emergency department staff. In practice, this takes time. As prompt chemoprophylaxis can limit the spread of pertussis (2), your priority should be to consider initiating this to eligible patients in the bay. The IPCT will also ensure correct isolation measures have been implemented to protect staff and other patients (3).

Pertussis is a notifiable disease in England and Wales (4). The public health department have already been informed and they will trace contacts outside the hospital to consider if chemoprophylaxis is required.

It is important to complete a clinical incident form so this incident can be logged, to help identify how this can be prevented from happening again.

Other important management steps include:

- Creating a safe environment for other patients and staff exposed
- Informing the consultant at the next appropriate opportunity
- Open communication with relatives of other patients in that bay
- Clear documentation in clinical notes

What happens to clinical incident forms once they have been completed?
Patient safety incidents are any unintended or unexpected incidents which could have, or did, lead to harm of one or more patients (5).

You will need to document:

- Location, date and time of the incident
- Description of the incident, including who was involved and affected
- The outcome to the person involved and what treatment was given
- Any other immediate action taken including the names of senior staff involved
- Any remedial action to minimise risk of recurrence
- The severity of the incident

The National Patient Safety Agency manages clinical incidents reported in England and Wales. These are logged on a national database called the National Reporting and Learning System (NRLS). The NRLS will report all serious incidents resulting in death or severe harm to the Care Quality Commission. In Scotland, incidents are logged using a Datix form online.

When an incident is logged, a Root Cause Analysis investigation then takes place locally. The purpose is to explore the contributing factors which compromised patient safety, how and why they occurred and identify areas of change to prevent them from occurring again, for example by developing a set of recommendations.

Human Factors

It is important to acknowledge the universal nature of human fallibility and inevitability of error, even in the best organisations (6). The understanding of human factors is crucial to optimise patient safety by enabling healthcare workers to consider what affects behaviour and performance in the workforce and to reduce risk of error to a minimum. Human factors are defined as 'environmental, organisational and job factors, and human and individual characteristics which influence behaviour at work in a way which can affect health and safety' (7).

Consider the many factors which may have contributed to this scenario:

Personal: It was a busy shift. Were you tired? Had you eaten lunch? Were you stressed about managing your workload? Were you worried about the patient you were performing the procedure puncture on? Was it a difficult procedure?

Task related: Did you know how to act on this result? If not, do you know how to find out? Do you know what guidelines to use? Do you have facilities to look them up?

Situational: Did you realise the impact of potential pertussis exposure on the other patients? Perhaps you could have asked the support worker to ask the laboratory to bleep back in 10-15 minutes time?

Organisational: Should the microbiology laboratory only release results to the doctor required to act on them? Could you have asked the support worker to explain you were completing a sterile procedure and could they bleep back in 10 minutes time? Could the result have been communicated to the nurse in charge as well? Would the laboratory also report these results automatically to infection control? Do you have a comprehensive handover to ensure all results get chased and acted on?

In this scenario, while there were a number of contributing factors, ineffective communication was the most significant. The result could have been communicated to a trained nurse or doctor able to deal with it, the staff member could have waited until the doctor had completed the procedure and communicated to the nurse in charge, and the nurse assisting the doctor could have ensured the result was communicated at nursing handover. The doctor allowed the support worker to interrupt a procedure instead of asking for information to be relayed later, and the doctor did not communicate the result to the nursing staff. This is effectively illustrated using the Swiss Cheese Model (5) with each slice of cheese representing a barrier between harm and the patient. The holes in the slices represent weaknesses in individual parts of the system. When all these holes line up, the harm reaches the patient.

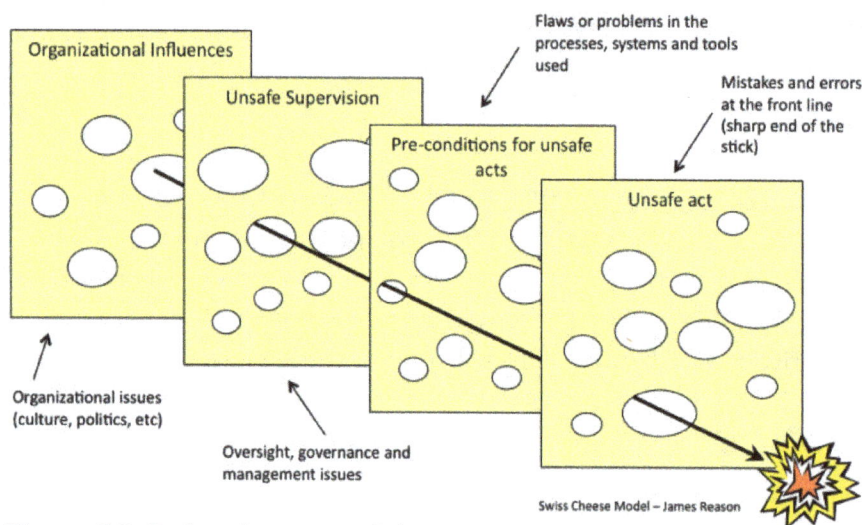

Figure 3.1: Swiss cheese model

Syllabus Mapping

Patient Safety and Clinical Governance

- Know the role of patient safety and clinical governance in safe healthcare delivery

- Be able to describe the impact of human factors on delivering safe clinical care

- Know how to exchange information in a timely manner to establish a shared understanding among appropriate members of the team

- Know the main routes of transmission of hospital acquired infections and their prevention

- Understand the factors that drive pandemic/epidemic infections and appreciate how this is used in clinical practice to prevent them

References

1. Jenkinson D. Natural course of 500 consecutive cases of whooping cough: a general practice population study. BMJ 1995;310(6975):299-302

2. Public Health Management of Pertussis. HPA Guidelines for the Public Health Management of Pertussis Incidents in Healthcare Settings. Health Protection Agency. 2012

3. Health protection legislation (England) guidance. Department of Health. Health Protection Agency. 2010.

4. Pertussis: guidance, data and analysis. Public Health England. 2014 https://www.gov.uk/government/collections/pertussis-guidance-data-and-analysis (accessed April 2016).

5. Reason J. Human error: models and management. BMJ 2000; 320 (7237): 768-770

6. Reducing error and influencing behaviour, HSG 48. Health and Safety Executive 2nd ed. 1999 page 2

7. Infection control precautions to minimise transmission of acute respiratory tract infections in healthcare settings. Public Health England. London. 2015

Further Reading

National Patient Safety Agency:
http://www.nrls.npsa.nhs.uk/home/ (accessed April 2016)
http://www.scottishpatientsafetyprogramme.scot.nhs.uk/about-us

Human Factors:
www.hse.gov.uk/humanfactors
http://www.who.int/patientsafety/research/methods_measures/human_factors/human_factors_review.
pdf?ua=1

Chapter 4: Wet, wet, wet
Dr Louise Oni

4

You are seeing patients in the emergency department. Your next patient is a 7 year old boy with a 24 hour history of high fever, vomiting, dysuria and enuresis. Since the age of 3 years he has had several episodes of high fever that have been unexplained and managed at home. He has a past history of a proven urinary tract infection (UTI) 6 months ago that was managed within primary care. He is developmentally appropriate and toilet trained during the daytime. He does however wet the bed most nights, passing a large volume of urine that doesn't wake him up.

On examination he weighs 12 kg (0.4^{th} centile) and is 92 cm tall (0.4^{th} centile). He is pale and febrile with a temperature of 39^0C. His blood pressure is 121/78 mmHg. Examination of his abdomen is normal except for some left sided flank tenderness. He has normal male genitalia and bilateral descended testes. Urine dipstick testing is positive for nitrites (+), leucocytes (3+), glucose (1+) and protein (1+)

Q1. What is the most important next test?

A.   Blood culture
B.   Blood glucose
C.   C reactive protein
D.   Full blood count
E.   Urine microscopy and culture

Q2. Following initiation of treatment which is the next investigation to be requested?

A.   24-hour blood pressure monitoring
B.   Dimercaptosuccinic acid (DMSA) scan
C.   Micturating cystourethrogram
D.   Renal ultrasound scan
E.   Urine protein:creatinine ratio

Following discharge he is seen in the out-patient clinic. During the clinic you also see 3 children with enuresis.

The following are potential management strategies:

A.   Alarm system
B.   Anti-cholinergic medication
C.   Bladder training
D.   Desmopressin medication
E.   Laxatives
F.   Lifting a sleeping child
G.   No intervention
H.   Reduce fluid intake during the evening
I.   Referral to tertiary specialist
J.   Tricyclic medication

For each of the following scenarios, choose the single most appropriate management option:

Q3a. A 5 year old girl with recurrent UTIs and poor growth who has daytime dribbling of urine and nocturnal enuresis.

Q3b. A 9 year old girl who has recently developed straining for her bowel openings with daytime frequency of urination and also has episodes of nocturnal enuresis occurring approximately once a month.

Q3c. A 7 year old boy who has been dry at daytime since the age of 2 years but who continues to have nocturnal enuresis every night and would like to be dry for a school camping trip in 2 months.

Answers and Rationale

Q1.   **E: Urine microscopy and culture**
Q2.   **D: Renal ultrasound scan**
Q3a.   **I: Referral to tertiary specialist**
Q3b.   **E: Laxatives**
Q3c.   **D: Desmopressin medication**

A child with a UTI will present with different symptoms depending on their age and stage of development. A toilet-trained or school age child will generally have similar symptoms to that of an adult with a UTI, including dysuria, frequency, pain and fever (1). Younger children may just have isolated fever or abdominal pain. The management of UTIs in children is in part dependent on the organism isolated on urine microscopy especially in children who have had a history of previous infections, therefore the urine microscopy and culture should be the next investigation to be performed. Most infections are caused by E coli organisms (2).

The following are risk factors for UTI that may indicate serious underlying pathology:

- poor urine flow
- history suggesting previous UTI or confirmed previous UTI
- recurrent fever of uncertain origin
- antenatally-diagnosed renal abnormality
- family history of VUR or renal disease
- constipation

- dysfunctional voiding
- enlarged bladder
- abdominal mass
- evidence of spinal lesion
- poor growth
- high blood pressure

Due to several risk factors the first case warrants further renal imaging. The best next test would be to perform a renal ultrasound scan as the patient has had recurrent UTIs and has risk factors for underlying pathology (recurrent fever of unknown origin, dysfunctional voiding, poor growth, high blood pressure). Table 4.1 summarises the age and indication for investigations. An ultrasound scan would determine the anatomy, size and shape of the kidneys (small kidneys indicate chronic disease, obstructions can be identified and irregular kidney shape may represent renal scars or current pyelonephritis). A DMSA scan is also indicated, as this is the best investigation to check for renal scarring, however it is better if this is performed 4-6 months after the acute infection to reduce the rate of false positive findings.

	Responds well to treatment*	Atypical UTI	Recurrent UTI
Child aged <6 months			
Ultrasound during acute period	No	Yes	Yes
Ultrasound within 6 weeks	Yes	No	No
DMSA 4-6 months	No	Yes	Yes
MCUG	No	Yes	Yes
Child aged 6 months to 3 years			
Ultrasound during acute period	No	Yes	No
Ultrasound within 6 weeks	No	No	Yes
DMSA 4-6 months	No	Yes	Yes
MCUG	No	No	No
Child aged over 3 years			
Ultrasound during acute period	No	Yes	No
Ultrasound within 6 weeks	No	No	Yes
DMSA 4-6 months	No	No	Yes
MCUG	No	No	No

Table 4.1: The child's age and characteristics of the urinary tract infection determine further investigations (2)

within 48 hours Abbreviations: UTI urinary tract infection; DMSA dimercaptosuccinic acid scan; MCUG micturating cystourethrogram

Bedwetting (nocturnal enuresis) is a common and distressing condition. The prevalence of bedwetting decreases with age, with wetting less than 2 nights a week having a prevalence of approximately 20% at 4.5 years and 8% at 9.5 years (3). More frequent bedwetting is less common and has a prevalence of 8% at 4.5 years and 1.5% at 9.5 years. Bedwetting that occurs every night is classed as severe and this is less likely to resolve spontaneously than infrequent bedwetting.

There are two kinds of enuresis: primary and secondary. Someone with primary enuresis has wet the bed since he or she was a baby. Secondary enuresis is a condition that develops at least 6 months — or often several years — after a person has learned to control his or her bladder. Secondary nocturnal enuresis accounts for about one quarter of children with bedwetting. Triggers for secondary enuresis include UTIs, diabetes mellitus, constipation, polyuric renal disease, behavioural changes or emotional events (4). Constipation is commonly associated also. A focused history is important and should determine whether these triggers are present (Table 4.2). A large volume of urine in the first few hours of the night is typical of bedwetting without any underlying renal abnormality. Symptoms suggestive of underlying renal or systemic pathology such as poor growth, recurrent infections or haematuria, demand referral to a specialist (3). Daytime symptoms may indicate a bladder disorder such as overactive bladder.

Questions to Ask When Taking the History of a Child with Bed-Wetting
Pattern of bedwetting
How many nights a week does bedwetting occur? How many times a night does bedwetting occur? Does there seem to be a large amount of urine? At what times of night does bedwetting occur? Does the child or young person wake up after bedwetting?
Daytime symptoms
Does the child or young person need to pass urine frequently (>7 times) or infrequently (<4 times) during the day? Does the child or young person need to pass urine urgently during the day? Is the child or young person wetting during the day? Does the child or young person have abdominal straining when passing urine or a poor urinary stream? Does the child or young person have pain passing urine?
Toileting patterns
Does the child or young person avoid using certain toilets, such as school toilets? Does the child or young person go to the toilet more or less often than his or her peers? Do daytime symptoms happen only in certain situations?
Fluid intake
How much does the child or young person drink during the day? Are they drinking less because of the bedwetting? Are the parents or carers restricting drinks because of the bedwetting?

Table 4.2: Questions to ask when taking the history in a child with bed-wetting (3)

There are several interventions that can assist in the management of bedwetting. Alarms will signal when they detect the first sign of urine and they have a high long-term success rate but can take several months before they demonstrate any difference. They also demand a commitment from the child and their family as they can be very disruptive. Lifting children to go to the toilet is sometimes used by parents to avoid changing the bedding however as it is done when they are still asleep it has no benefit on improving the long term prognosis (3). With regards to medications, Desmopressin is a synthetic replacement for Vasopressin, the hormone that reduces urine production. It is effective for rapid, short-term results. Anti-cholinergic medications can be useful for children with symptoms suggestive of bladder instability (daytime symptoms, urgency, small volume capacity, frequent urination) and tricyclic medications (such as desipramine or imipramine) can be used for nocturnal symptoms, their exact mechanism of action is not known. Bladder training encourages increasing the oral fluid intake during the daytime to improve the overall bladder capacity and reducing fluid intake in the evenings to reduce nocturnal volumes of urine. This is good practice for all patients. Laxatives are essential in cases where constipation may be aggravating the bladder symptoms.

Syllabus Mapping

Behavioural Medicine/Psychiatry

• Understand the principles of managing common emotional and behavioural problems such as temper tantrums, breath-holding attacks, sleep problems, feeding problems, the crying baby, oppositional behaviour, enuresis and encoporesis, excessive water drinking, school refusal, bullying and chronic fatigue syndrome and know when to refer

Nephro-urology

• Know the manifestations of acute and chronic renal disease

• Know the manifestations and management of urinary tract infections in different age groups

• Know the principles of managing enuresis

References and Further Reading

1. Stein R, Dogan HS, Hoebeke P, Kočvara R, Nijman RJ, Radmayr C, Tekgül S. Urinary tract infections in children: EAU/ESPU guidelines. European urology. 2015 Mar 31;67(3):546-58

2. Baumer JH, Jones RW. Urinary tract infection in children, National Institute for Health and Clinical Excellence. Archives of disease in childhood-Education & practice edition. 2007 Dec 1;92(6):189-92

3. Nocturnal Enuresis. The management of bedwetting in children and young people. National Clinical Guideline Centre (UK). London: Royal College of Physicians. 2010 Oct

4. Nunes VD, O'Flynn N, Evans J, Sawyer L. Management of bedwetting in children and young people: summary of NICE guidance. BMJ: British Medical Journal. 2010 Oct 30;341(7779):936-8

Chapter 5: A noisy 3 year old
Dr Elliott Ridgeon and Dr Anna Mathew

5

You are on call and are called to the emergency department to review Jaz, an 18 month old boy. When you arrive he is sitting up in bed, breathing noisily with an occasionally harsh cough. His mother tells you that he has been unwell for the last few days with a cough, he hasn't eaten much and has not been keen to play. Jaz is reluctant to interact with you but when he does talk to his mother you notice his voice is hoarse.

His temperature is 37.7°C, heart rate 105/minute, respiratory rate 41/minute and oxygen saturations 96% in air. On examination he is using his accessory muscles to breathe and has harsh, transmitted sounds on inspiration but no wheeze or crackles. Cardiovascular examination is normal and his capillary refill time is 2 seconds centrally.

Q1. Which organism is the most likely cause of this presentation?

A. Corynebacterium diphtheria
B. Haemophilus influenzae
C. Parainfluenza
D. RSV (Respiratory Syncitial Virus)
E. Streptococcus pneumonia

Q2. Which one of the following is the mainstay of management in this case?

A. Intravenous cephalosporin
B. Intravenous fluids
C. Nebulised adrenaline
D. Oral steroids
E. Urgent bronchoscopy

Q3. Which one of the following investigations should be undertaken?

A. Blood samples (full blood count, urea, electrolytes)
B. Frontal neck X ray
C. MRI neck
D. No immediate investigation necessary
E. Throat swabs

Answers and Rationale

Q1.   C: Parainfluenza
Q2.   D: Oral steroids
Q3.   D: No immediate investigation necessary

Management of stridor of any cause should be based around the emergency assessment principles of ABC (Airway, Breathing, and Circulation). Paediatricians and Emergency/General Physicians should have a low threshold for referral and escalation to colleagues in anaesthetics, critical care and ENT surgery. Examination of the mouth/airway should be avoided without the presence of an airway-competent doctor, so as to avoid distressing the child, irritating the airway and risking complete obstruction. Jaz is most likely to have croup (laryngo-tracheobronchitis). Croup is a diagnosis made clinically with classical features including onset of symptoms over 24-72h, a harsh "barking" cough, stridor and a hoarse voice. Importantly, the child does not have features of some of the more worrying differential diagnoses (drooling, "toxic" and unwell appearance), as outlined in boxes 1 and 2. Croup is commonly caused by parainfluenza virus. Influenza A/B, RSV and rhinovirus can also be implicated (1). Bacterial infection (bacterial tracheitis) can arise secondarily, and is acute and potentially life-threatening. This is usually caused by H influenzae, S aureus or S pneumoniae (2). Immunisation has now made severe infective causes of stridor rare (notably epiglottitis and diphtheria), but these must be considered in a differential diagnosis. This is particularly important if there is a suspicion that the child may not be up to date with vaccinations. Foreign body inhalation remains relatively common, and can be life-threatening, but patients will usually present with a history of a witnessed inhalation event, and without the prominent hoarseness and cough.

Box 1 – Differential Diagnosis of Stridor in Children	
Infective	Croup
	Epiglottitis
	Bacterial tracheitis
	Retropharyngeal abscess
	Diphtheria
Inflammatory	Anaphylaxis
	Hereditary angioedema
Other	Foreign body inhalation
	Tracheomalacia

Box 2 – Croup versus Epiglottitis	
Croup	**Epiglottitis**
Slower onset	Rapid onset
Prominent "barking" cough	Cough not prominent
Not drooling, able to swallow, hoarse voice	Drooling, unable to swallow or talk
Does not appear "toxic" or profoundly unwell	Sick appearing child, unwell

Given the potential threat to the airway, distressing the child with invasive investigation (e.g. needles for blood sampling, throat swabs) is unwise, as is moving the child around the hospital to obtain imaging.

However, if there is diagnostic uncertainty, and a more sinister problem is suspected, then laboratory tests and radiology may be required (e.g. retropharyngeal abscess, foreign body inhalation). If a frontal neck x-ray is performed the characteristic "steeple" sign – narrowing of the subglottic space such that the lower airway resembles a church steeple - may be seen in croup. Note that the absence of this sign does not rule out the diagnosis of croup. Patients with epiglottitis may have a thickened epiglottis seen on x-ray, while those with a retropharyngeal abscess may have a soft tissue bulge on the posterior wall of the pharynx. Irregular tracheal mucosa, sometimes with strands across the lumen, can indicate bacterial tracheitis (3).

Recurrent croup (defined as two or more croup episodes in a year) should be viewed as a separate clinical entity from viral croup, and does require investigation for a cause. If atopy is ruled out as a possible explanation, direct laryngo-tracheo-bronchoscopy is essential, as anatomical airway problems are a significant cause of recurrent croup. Imaging with x-ray, CT or MR can also help in cases of suspected airway compression due to extra-tracheal mass (e.g. tumour, abscess) (4).

Oral glucocorticoids have been shown to relieve symptoms of croup, reduce length of hospital stay, and need for admission/re-admission (5). Dexamethasone may be superior to prednisolone in reducing admission rates, but evidence is conflicting (6-7). Oral administration is equally effective when compared to IM or nebulised steroids (Budesonide), and has the advantage of causing less distress to the child. If the child is unable to swallow, then IM can be used, but this symptom in itself may suggest an alternative, more sinister diagnosis.

Nebulised adrenaline can be a helpful adjunct to steroids in severe cases. It is important to be mindful of the short duration of action which may result in a short lived improvement and rebound of symptoms. There is also the risk of tachyarrhythmia.

If superimposed bacterial infection is suspected, antibiotics should be considered, along with other resuscitation (e.g. fluids) as needed. Humidified air has no role in treating croup. Evidence for use of heliox is currently inconclusive (8).

Management of croup can be guided by assessment of severity, using the categories shown in box 3, and strategies in box 4.

Box 3 – Determining Severity of Croup		
Mild	**Moderate**	**Severe**
Occasional barking cough	Frequent barking cough	Frequent barking cough
No stridor at rest	Some stridor at rest	Prominent stridor at rest
No / mild accessory muscle use and suprasternal/intercostal recession	Some accessory muscle use, with suprasternal/intercostal recession	Marked difficulty in breathing, with suprasternal/intercostal recession
Child appears well, eating, drinking, playing	Child can be placated, will reluctantly engage	Some distress and agitation, progressing to lethargy if hypoxic

Box 4 – Management Strategies for Croup (3)		
Mild	**Moderate**	**Severe**
Oral dexamethasone Educate parents about signs of respiratory distress and when to seek further help Discharge home	Oral dexamethasone Observe for improvement: If better within approximately 4h, treat as mild (discharge home). If no improvement, consider secondary measures and escalation as per severe case.	Oral dexamethasone Nebulised Budesonide Nebulised adrenaline Oxygen – use "blow-by" technique of holding mask near face to minimise distress Admit to hospital, escalate to paediatric ICU if worsening

Syllabus Mapping

Respiratory Medicine with ENT

- Know the causes of stridor and the principles of management

References and Further Reading

1. Miller EK, Gebretsadik T, Carroll KN, Dupont WD, Mohamed YA, Morin LL, Heil L, Minton PA, Woodward K, Liu Z, Hartert TV. Viral Etiologies of Infant Bronchiolitis, Croup, and Upper Respiratory Illness during Four Consecutive Years. The Pediatric infectious disease journal. 2013 Sep;32(9)

2. Zoorob R, Sidani M, Murray J. Croup: an overview. Am Fam Physician. 2011 May 1;83(9):1067-73

3. Bjornson, Candice L., and David W. Johnson. "Croup in Children." CMAJ : Canadian Medical Association Journal 185.15 (2013): 1317–1323. PMC. Web. 16 Dec. 2016

4. Joshi V, Malik V, Mirza O, Kumar BN. Fifteen-minute consultation: structured approach to management of a child with recurrent croup. Archives of disease in childhood-Education & practice edition. 2013 Nov 14:edpract-2013

5. Russell KF, Liang Y, O'Gorman K, Johnson DW, Klassen TP. Glucocorticoids for croup. The Cochrane Library. 2011 Jan 1.

6. Sparrow A, Geelhoed G. Prednisolone versus dexamethasone in croup: a randomised equivalence trial. Archives of disease in childhood. 2006 Jul 1;91(7):580-3

7. Fifoot AA, Ting J. Comparison between single-dose oral prednisolone and oral dexamethasone in the treatment of croup: A randomized, double-blinded clinical trial. Emergency Medicine Australasia. 2007 Feb 1;19(1):51-8

8. Vorwerk C, Coats T. Heliox for croup in children. The Cochrane Library. 2010 Jan 1

Chapter 6: "Is it a tumour?"
Dr Louise Cutts

6

You see Melody in clinic, a 4 month old girl with a bright red, well-demarcated nodule on the left chest. This wasn't present at birth but appeared at a month old and has been increasing in size. It doesn't appear to trouble her but her parents are particularly concerned by its appearance. They have been told by her GP that this is a harmless birthmark called a haemangioma but have asked the appointment to be brought forward as a neighbour had said it is a tumour.

Q1. What is the best management at this stage?

A. Intravenous Propranolol
B. Observation. No active intervention is currently indicated
C. Oral corticosteroid
D. Oral Propranolol
E. Refer for laser treatment

Q2. What is the best information to tell the parents at this stage?

A. Bleeding is a common complication
B. Laser therapy is likely to be needed in the future
C. The haemangioma is likely to continue enlarging and then involute
D. There will be no need for any active intervention in the future
E. Ulceration is a common complication

Q3. Which is the most important investigation to be requested in an infant with >10 haemangiomas?

A. Abdominal ultrasound scan
B. Clotting studies
C. ECG
D. Echocardiogram
E. Full blood count

Answers and Rational

Q1. B: Observation. No active intervention is currently indicated
Q2. C: The haemangioma is likely to continue enlarging and then involute
Q3. A: Abdominal ultrasound scan

Haemangiomas are the most common tumours of infancy. Other common paediatric skin lesions are listed in (Table 1). Haemangiomas are benign tumours of vascular endothelium and can be superficial, deep or mixed. Superficial haemangiomas appear as vivid red, well-demarcated plaques or nodules. Deep haemangiomas are skin-coloured or less well defined. Mixed haemangiomas have characteristics of both.

Up to half of haemangiomas are present at birth with the rest usually becoming apparent in the first month of life. Pre-cursor lesions can appear as a blanched macule, erythematous or telangectatic patch or a bruised-like area. They undergo a proliferative growth phase which generally lasts for 6-9 months, but can be longer in deep haemangiomas. This is followed by stabilisation and then spontaneous involution. As the haemangioma involutes the bright red colour is replaced by a purple hue which in turn this becomes grey centrally and then peripherally. The lesion then flattens and softens (1).

In most cases haemangiomas have a benign self-limiting course and reassurance is all that is required. However complications such as ulceration, bleeding and life-altering disfigurement prompt a need for intervention. Profuse bleeding is an uncommon complication and can usually be managed with light pressure to the area. Ulceration tends to occur during rapid proliferation. It can cause considerable pain, infection and also result in scar formation.

Haemangiomas that compromise vital organ function such as those situated near the eye, nose, ears, lips, airway and anogenital tract also warrant intervention. Segmental haemangiomas in a cervicofacial, mandibular or "beard" distribution can be associated with airway haemangiomas. Infants with involved airway haemangiomas can present with stridor in the first 6-12 weeks of life; this is most common during the proliferative growth phase (3). Multiple or segmental haemangiomas may signify additional internal lesions of the liver, brain, gastrointestinal tract and airway with the liver being the most common location for visceral involvement (2). These infants should have a liver ultrasound to detect the presence of haemangiomas.

The non-selective β-antagonist propranolol is first-line treatment for infantile haemangiomas. It is thought to exert its effects through a variety of mechanisms such as vasoconstriction, the blocking of pro-angiogenic signals such as vascular endothelial growth factor and apoptosis (4,5). Before initiation of propranolol a full history and examination should take place, focusing on signs and symptoms of cardiac and pulmonary disease. Children with bradycardia, history of arrhythmia or a family history of congenital heart condition should also undergo an ECG and echocardiogram. Contraindications for propranolol therapy include cardiogenic shock, sinus, bradycardia, hypotension, greater than first-degree heart block, greater than first-degree heart block, bronchial hypersensitivity and hypersensitivity to propranolol.

Aquired melanocytic naevus	These are moles which appear after birth as flat lesions and may become elevated. They vary in colour from pink or flesh-coloured to various shades of brown.
Congenital melanocytic naevus	Occur due to a proliferation of benign melanocytes which are present at birth or shortly after birth. They can be classified as small <1.5cm, medium 1.5-20cm, large >20cm and giant >40cm.
Dermal melanocytic naevus	Appear blue in colour due to the presence of melanin in the dermis. Types include: • Common blue naevi – raised, dome shaped blue lesions. • Naevus of Ota – in the distribution of the opthalmic and axillary branch of the trigeminal nerve. • Naevus of Ito – on the scapula area • Mongolion blue spot – blue-grey marking often occurring on the lumbar-sacral region
Granuloma annulare	Characterised by annular dermal plaques, common in childhood. Thought to be due to a delayed hypersensitivity reaction.
Halo naevus	Melanocytic naevus with a white ring or halo of depigmentation around it. Common in childhood and sometimes associated with vitiligo.
Milia	Appear as superficial pearly-white papules which are tiny cysts filled with keratin. Most commonly arise on the face and affect 40-50% of newborn babies.
Molluscum contagiosum	Dome-shaped flesh coloured papules, often associated with atopic eczema. They are due to the pox virus and are usually self-limiting.
Sebaceous naevus	A type of epidermal naevus which often presents as a yellow-orange hairless patch or plaque. Present from birth and most commonly found on the scalp and face due to the abundant sebaceous glands in these areas.
Spitz naevus	Solitary dome-shaped red or reddish-brown papule or nodule. 70% diagnosed in the first 20 years of life. May grow up to 1-2cm in diameter. Difficult to predict the outcome, therefore excision recommended.

Table 6.1: Common paediatric skin lesions

PHACE syndrome is characterised by a large segmental haemangioma, usually on the face or head. It is a neurocutaneous syndrome with a number of associations. Any infant where PHACE syndrome is suspected should undergo MRI/MRA brain and neck, cardiac and ophthalmic assessment.

P   Posterior fossa brain malformations
H   Haemangiomas, particularly large segmental facial lesions
A   Arterial anomalies
C   Cardiac anomalies and coarctation of the aorta
E   Eye and endocrine abnormalities

Patients with suspected PHACE syndrome who are commencing on propranolol require a pre-treatment magnetic resonance angiogram to detect any underlying arterial anomalies because of the increased risk of stroke. These patients should be managed closely within a multidisciplinary team involving dermatology and cardiology. Thyroid function tests are necessary in the presence of liver, parotid or very large haemangiomas to detect hypothyroidism and in PHACE syndrome to exclude congenital hypothyroidism. Serious adverse side-effects include bradycardia, hypotension, hyperkalaemia, bronchospasm and hypoglycaemia (6). Education of parents and carers should involve explaining the natural course, potential complications, indications for treatment, treatment benefits and risks and also managing expectations. A leaflet with a direct contact number for the responsible team should also be issued.

Syllabus Mapping

Dermatology

- Be able to assess simple birth marks such as strawberry naevi and Mongolian blue spots and refer when appropriate

- Understand the emotional impact of severe dermatological problems

References and Further Reading

1. Bruckner AL and Frieden IJ. Infantile Haemangiomas and Other Vascular Tumours. In: Irvine AD, Hoeger PH, Yan AC eds. Harper's Textbook of Pediatric Dermatology. Third Edition. Chichester: Wiley-Blackwell 2011

2. Darrow DH, Greene AK, Mancini AJ, Nopper AJ, Antaya RJ, Cohen B, Drolet BA, Fay A, Fishman SJ, Friedlander SF, Ghali FE. Diagnosis and Management of Infantile Hemangioma. Pediatrics. 2015 Oct 1;136(4):e1060-104

3. Drolet BA, Esterly NB, Frieden IJ. Hemangiomas in children. New England Journal of Medicine. 1999 Jul 15;341(3):173-81

4. Storch CH, Hoeger PH. Propranolol for infantile haemangiomas: insights into the molecular mechanisms of action. British Journal of Dermatology. 2010 Aug 1;163(2):269-74

5. Solman L, Murabit A, Gnarra M, Harper JI, Syed SB, Glover M. Propranolol for infantile haemangiomas: single centre experience of 250 cases and proposed therapeutic protocol. Archives of disease in childhood. 2014 Dec 1;99(12):1132-6

6. Drolet BA, Frommelt PC, Chamlin SL, Haggstrom A, Bauman NM, Chiu YE, Chun RH, Garzon MC, Holland KE, Liberman L, MacLellan-Tobert S. Initiation and use of propranolol for infantile hemangioma: report of a consensus conference. Pediatrics. 2013 Jan 1;131(1):128-40

Chapter 7: A waiting room full of hot children
Dr Jim Gould

You are back working in the emergency department. As you start your shift the nurse practitioner hands over the following 3 children who she has reviewed and wants you to see.

Sam is a 4 week old baby boy with a 4 day history of irritability, fever and not moving his left arm as usual. On examination his temperature is 38.5°C, heart rate 150/minute, blood pressure 65/45 mmHg and capillary refill time <2 seconds. No rash or bruising is seen. He has no cardiac murmurs and his chest is clear. His abdomen is soft with no guarding, but his spleen tip is just palpable. There is a warm swelling of the left upper arm which appears to be tender.

Jack is a 4 year old boy with a 48 hour history of lethargy and pyrexia. Yesterday he complained of a sore right knee and was not keen to walk. He has had all his routine childhood immunisations to date. Examination shows a swollen and tender right knee, with a few scattered non-blanching spots on his trunk, most > 3mm in size. His heart rate is 140/minute, blood pressure is 65/45mmHg, central capillary refill time 4 seconds and respiratory rate is 30/minute.

Aisha is a 4 month old baby with a 2 day history of poor feeding, non-projectile vomiting for the last 24 hours and lethargy. On examination she has a temperature of 38.8°C. Her heart rate is 145/minute, blood pressure 80/55mmHg with a respiratory rate of 35/minute. She is tender on palpation of her right flank. Her anterior fontanelle is normal, there are no cardiac murmurs and her chest is clear to auscultation.

Q1. In what order would you review these children?

A. Aisha, Jack, Sam
B. Jack, Aisha, Sam
C. Jack, Sam, Aisha
D. Sam, Aisha, Jack
E. Sam, Jack, Aisha

Q2. Here is a list of bacteria that can produce sepsis in young children:

A. Escherichia coli
B. Haemophilus influenzae type
C. Listeria monocytogenes
D. Mycoplasma pneumoniae
E. Neisseria meningitides
F. Pseudomonas aeruginosa
G. Staphylococcus aureus
H. Streptococcus agalactiae (Group B Strep.)
I. Streptococcus pyogenes (Group A Strep.)
J. Streptococcus pneumoniae (Pneumococcus)

Chose the most likely bacterium causing sepsis in:

Q2a. Sam

Q2b. Jack

Q2c. Aisha

Answers and Rationale

Q1. **C: Jack, Sam, Aisha**
Q2a **H: Streptococcus agalactiae (Group B Strep.)**
Q2b. **E: Neisseria meningitides**
Q2c. **A: Escherichia coli**

You will be frequently asked to undertake the assessment and initial management of feverish illness in children under 5 years of age. Systematic reviews of evidence have led to the publication of a number of guidelines on the subject, most importantly the NICE guideline (1). The Traffic Light system for identifying risk of serious illness based on clinical signs and symptoms has been adopted in these guidelines. The "Red –High Risk symptoms and signs are below: (Table 7.1).

Using these guidelines allows you to prioritise the order in which you would see the children. Both Sam (Temp ≥ 38°C less than 3 months) and Jack (non-blanching rash) have "Red – high risk " signs however Jack's signs of cardiovascular compromise (tachycardia and reduced capillary refill time) and likely underlying diagnosis of meningococcal sepsis necessitate him being seen and treated urgently, before Sam. Aisha also requires prompt review and treatment and one would call for assistance in managing this situation.

	Red - high risk symptoms and signs	
Colour (of skin, lips or tongue)	• Pale/mottled/ashen/blue	
Activity	• No response to social cues • Appears ill to a healthcare professional	• Unrousable/drowsy Weak, high-pitched or continuous cry
Respiratory	• Grunting • Tachypnoea	• RR >60 breaths/minute • Moderate or severe chest in-drawing
Circulation/ hydration	• Reduced skin turgor	
Other	• Age <3 months temp. ≥38°C • Non-blanching rash • Bulging fontanelle • Neck stiffness	• Status epilepticus • Focal neurological signs • Focal seizures

Table 7.1: NICE: Traffic light system for identifying risk of serious illness in Children < 5 years with fever

With likely sepsis in a young child it is important to know not only that antibiotics are indicated and need to be administered with urgency, but also the most likely infecting organism so that the most appropriate antibiotic and other therapies (such as fluids, inotropic agents) can be administered promptly, and appropriate investigations undertaken to confirm the diagnosis (Table 7.2).

Late onset Group B Strep. Infection

A four week old baby with a swelling of the upper arm has either had a humeral fracture, developed a tumour or has localised osteomyelitis, with possible septic arthritis of the shoulder joint. With Sam's presentation and fever, the last of these possibilities is the most likely. An X-ray is likely to assist in distinguishing between these diagnoses even though osteomyelitis may result in no changes on early imaging. Osteomyelitis at around this age is very likely to relate to late onset (>7 days and <90 days of age) Group B streptococcal infection. In contrast to early onset disease maternal obstetric complications are not risk factors for the development of late onset disease. In addition, late onset disease is not prevented by antibiotics administered in labour may also not be as a result of vertical transmission. In this infant with fever and irritability, co-existing early meningitis is quite likely, so as part of the investigations (FBC, inflammatory markers, blood and urine culture) a lumbar puncture would be obligatory as long as the is stable enough for the procedure. Treatment with high dose systemic penicillin for a minimum of 3-4 weeks is required with the option of the addition of clindamycin or vancomycin (depending on organism sensitivity) for maximal antibiotic penetration into bone when treating bone/joint infection (2).

Meningococcal infection

The presence of non-blanching purpuric spots, especially >2mm diameter, even if only a few are present, should alert the examiner to the likelihood of a meningococcal infection. Other bacteria can occasionally produce purpura including *listeria* and *pneumococcus*, but this is rare, especially in this age group. In a fevered child this finding constitutes a medical emergency requiring immediate action as at times the disease process can advance within hours to widespread necrotic purpura and ecchymosis, associated with vascular collapse (3). Not all children conform to an identical disease pattern. Some children will develop an initial covert bacteraemia with spread of bacteria to the meninges, bone or joints and therefore develop focal disease (in this case a right septic arthritis of the knee) before developing further bacteraemic spread with evidence of scattered cutaneous lesions. Such children can go on to develop a full-blown septicaemia and need to be assessed and monitored carefully. In Jack's case, the prolonged capillary refill time, tachycardia and low blood pressure suggest that a poorly compensated septicaemic shock is developing and urgent fluid replacement as well as high dose systemic antibiotics, oxygen and other supportive measures will be required.

The prevention of meningococcal disease in the UK has advanced recently with the introduction of the multicomponent protein meningococcal B vaccine to the routine infant immunisation schedule to complement conjugate meningococcal C vaccine and the quadrivalent polysaccharide vaccine covering capsular groups A,C,W and Y(available as both conjugated and non-conjugated vaccines). For further information and explanation of the use of these conjugated and non-conjugated vaccines see the "Green Book" (4).

Diagnosis	Symptoms and signs in conjunction with fever	
Meningococcal disease	Non-blanching rash, with 1 or more of the following: • an ill-looking child • lesions larger than 2 mm in diameter (purpura)	• capillary refill time of ≥3 seconds • neck stiffness
Bacterial meningitis	• Neck stiffness • Bulging fontanelle	• Decreased level of consciousness • Convulsive status epilepticus
Herpes simplex encephalitis	• Focal neurological signs • Focal seizures	• Decreased level of consciousness
Pneumonia	• Tachypnoea • Crackles in the chest • Nasal flaring	• Chest indrawing • Cyanosis • Oxygen saturation ≤95%
Urinary tract infection	• Vomiting • Poor feeding • Lethargy	• Irritability • Abdominal pain or tenderness • Urinary frequency or dysuria
Septic arthritis	• Swelling of a limb or joint • Not using an extremity	• Non-weight bearing
Kawasaki disease	Fever for more than 5 days and at least 4 of the following: • bilateral conjunctival injection • change in mucous membranes	• change in the extremities • polymorphous rash • cervical lymphadenopathy

Table 7.2: Summary table for symptoms and signs suggestive of specific diseases (adapted from NICE Guideline cg160 (2013)

E. Coli UTI

Any children presenting with relatively non-specific symptoms of poor feeding, occasional vomiting and lethargy may have a urine infection. Aisha has right flank tenderness suggesting the possibility of right renal pathology such as a pyelonephritis. It is important to differentiate children with symptoms merely suggesting cystitis from those with additional upper renal tract involvement as this may be a pointer to a renal tract abnormality allowing reflux. Obtaining an uncontaminated urine sample for investigation in a female infant can be difficult. A "clean catch" sample is regarded as best, but at times a supra-pubic aspiration (SPA) may need to be performed after ensuring that there is sufficient urine in the bladder by ultrasound examination. In children under the age of three years, urgent microscopy and culture of the urine is the preferred method for diagnosing a UTI rather than relying on dipstick analysis for leukocyte esterase and nitrites. In this case E.Coli is by far the most likely organism of those listed. Treatment pending culture and antibiotic sensitivity testing should be with a broad spectrum antibiotic with low resistance pattern such as co-amoxiclav for 7-10 days, given IV initially if not tolerated orally. Investigation of the infant's renal tract should be undertaken (5).

Syllabus Mapping

Infection, Immunology and Allergy

* Know about common infections of children in the UK and important worldwide infections, e.g. TB, HIV, hepatitis B, malaria, polio

* Be able to assess and manage a febrile child and have knowledge of current evidence based guidelines

* Know when antimicrobials are indicated

* Understand the normal patterns and frequency of infections in childhood

Nephro-urology

* Know the manifestations and management of urinary tract infections in different age groups

Neurology

* Know the likely causes and management of meningitis/encephalitis and altered consciousness

References and Further Reading

1. Fever in under 5s: assessment and initial management. NICE guidelines CG160. May 2013

2. Sass L. Group B streptococcal infections. Pediatrics in review/American Academy of Pediatrics. 2012 May; 33(5):219

3. Meningitis (bacterial) and meningococcal septicaemia in under 16s: recognition, diagnosis and management. NICE Guidelines CG102. June 2010

4. Department of Health (updated 2014) Immunisation against infectious disease [the 'Green book']. London: Chapter 22 Meningococcal

5. Urinary tract infection in under 16s: diagnosis and management. NICE Guidelines CG54. August 2007

Chapter 8: Planning for a good death
Dr Susie Holt and Mrs Lesley Fellows

8

Kevin is a 5 year old boy with mitochondrial respiratory chain deficiency, which is a life-limiting condition. He is likely to die during childhood. He was born at 27 weeks gestation and has chronic lung disease. He has significant global developmental delay, requires continuous invasive ventilation and is fed via a gastrostomy. He lives with his parents and has 2 siblings.

He has spent a lot of his life in hospital due to complications of his disease. When he is well he is mobile, communicates with Makaton sign language and attends a special needs school. Over the past few months he has had 3 acute admissions to hospital with respiratory symptoms including apnoea, difficulty maintaining saturations and associated bradycardia. This is a new development. Despite thorough investigation no reversible cause has been identified for these episodes that cause both Kevin and his family a lot of distress.

Q1. Which one of the following should be the focus of Kevin's future care plan?

A.   Acute management of each episode in hospital
B.   Admission to hospital for observation of episodes and further investigation
C.   End of life care
D.   No further treatment
E.   Palliative care

Q2. Which one of the following does an advanced care plan (ACP) _not_ include:

A.   Decision not to admit to a critical care area
B.   Decision to implement ceilings of care e.g. oral antibiotics but no intravenous antibiotic
C.   Details of professionals involved in patient care
D.   Instructions on where the body should be cared for after death
E.   Legally-binding "Do Not Resuscitate" order

Here is a list of providers of bereavement support:

A.   General Practitioner
B.   Hospice
C.   Hospital bereavement team
D.   Hospital Chaplain
E.   Hospital Consultant involved in child's care

F.   Hospital Psychologists
G.   Social Services
H.   Specialist charities e.g. Sands
I.   Telephone line e.g. Child Death Helpline
J.   Websites e.g. Together for Short Lives

Choose the most likely avenue of support given the different needs of the people affected:

Q3a. The family of a stillborn baby want a blessing for their infant

Q3b. A recently bereaved single mother wakes at 03:00 inconsolably crying

Q3c. The family of a child with terminal cancer wish to discuss the options to plan for his death

Answers and Rationale

Q1.   **E: Palliative care**
Q2.   **E: Legally-binding "Do Not Resuscitate" order**
Q3a.   **D: Hospital Chaplain**
Q3b.   **I: Telephone line e.g. Child Death Helpline**
Q3c.   **B: Hospice**

Palliative care for children and young people is an active and total approach to care from the point of diagnosis or recognition, embracing physical, emotional, social and spiritual elements through to death and beyond. It focuses on enhancement of quality of life for the child/young person and support for the family. It includes the management of distressing symptoms, provision of short respite breaks, and care through death and bereavement (1). A child does not need to be imminently dying to benefit from palliative care and frequently a palliative care journey will include several episodes of serious ill health where a child is sick enough that they might die, but they then recover and return to being clinically stable for a further period of time.

Kevin's new symptoms could potentially represent deterioration. This information was shared with the family but it is vital to acknowledge the uncertainty in predicting whether this deterioration would lead to a plateau in symptoms, a clinical improvement or move to end of life care and death. Acknowledging the concern of deterioration to the family enables further discussions focusing on planning Kevin's future care - a process known as advanced care planning. This falls under the umbrella term "palliative care".

An advanced care plan (ACP) is designed to communicate the health-care wishes of children who have chronic and life-limiting conditions. It sets out an agreed plan of care to be followed when a child's condition deteriorates. It provides a framework for both discussing and documenting the agreed wishes of a child and their parents for when the child develops potentially life-threatening complications. Where a child is considered to have capacity their views should be considered in the decision-making. The ACP is designed so that it can be used in all environments: home, hospital, school, hospice and respite care. It is also appropriate for use by the ambulance service. An ACP can be used as a resuscitation plan and/ or as an end-of-life care plan. It remains valid when parents or next of kin cannot be contacted but is not a legally binding document (2). Many areas around the UK are choosing to use a similar template for the ACP so that the document is widely recognised.

The ACP is a unique document to each child and family. It contains the diagnosis and an explanation of the how the illness affects the child including relevant past medical history. It includes any adjuncts the child requires (e.g. gastrostomy, non-invasive ventilation) and any relevant plans such as feeding plans. The family often like to include hints and tips on how to care for their child, particularly if they are non-verbal, for example what calms them down. Additionally, the family can choose to insert details of how to care for their child after death and any funeral plans.

In Kevin's ACP there should be details on how to manage his episodes of respiratory distress. This symptom is potentially life-threatening and if he did not respond to interventions then the clinical team would need to change the focus to end of life care. Therefore, his ACP needs to focus on both what to do if his saturations recover and also what to do if they don't – this is termed 'parallel planning.' Parallel plans for other anticipated symptoms are also considered and written down in advance e.g. how to treat infection, whether to care for a child in a critical care area. Parallel planning for life while also planning for deterioration or death allows a child's full potential to be achieved and primes the mobilisation of services and professionals when and where necessary (3). End of life care is part of palliative care but focuses on preparing for an anticipated death and managing the end stage of a terminal medical condition. This includes care during and around the time of death and immediately afterwards. An anticipatory symptom management plan (SMP), including prescribing, focuses on current and condition-specific likely symptoms at end of life and enables the clinical team delivering care to promote a 'good death' or more commonly 'the least bad death' from the family's point of view. The 6 key anticipated symptoms at end of life include: breathlessness, pain, terminal agitation/anxiety, nausea/vomiting, secretions and seizures. Management of all of these symptoms are integral to any SMP.

A comprehensive palliative care service requires a multidisciplinary team approach, involving health, social care, education and the voluntary sectors, mainly hospices. The first children's hospice opened in 1982 and there are now more than 40 in the UK. They offer a wide range of services including:
- 24 hour end of life care
- support for the entire family (including siblings, grandparents and the extended family)
- bereavement support
- 24 hour access to emergency care
- specialist short break care
- 24 hour telephone support
- practical help, advice and information
- provision of specialist therapies, including physiotherapy, play, complementary and music therapy
- provision of information, support, education and training to carers, where needed
- community-based teams offering many of the same services in the home environment

Caring for a technology-dependent child is physically, emotionally and financially challenging. Continuing health care funded packages, overseen by designated social workers, often support parents delivering the 24-hour care their child requires.

Palliative care also focuses on spiritual, social and emotional aspects of care for the patient, their family and carers. Kevin's family were able to access psychology services at the tertiary hospital and counselling services at the hospice. Exploring anticipatory grief often supports the post-bereavement process reducing complicated grief. Provision of play therapy, 1:1 counselling and peer group counselling is often offered through children's hospice services however other sources of psychological and bereavement support can be sourced through General Practice, tertiary centres and other charitable organisations including online resources such as Child Bereavement UK (4) and Winston's Wish (5). The Child Death Helpline, staffed by volunteers, offers telephone support to anyone affected by the death of a child.

Families may wish to engage with religious or spiritual leaders and many hospitals have a chaplaincy service with links to other religious leaders in the community. Some hospitals will also have a prayer room. In all care settings: hospitals, hospices or at home; families should be offered a blessing or prayers at the bedside as well as exploring their own belief's around death and dying. There may be specific support groups, for example "Children of Jannah" support Muslim families affected by bereavement, relevant to individual patients.

Exploring what is important to a child and family and supporting them to create lasting memories can help them achieve what can be described as a "good death". Collecting mementoes such as hand and foot prints locks of hair and photographs can help the bereavement process. There are many charities who grant children a 'wish', the memory of which the family will cherish forever.

Kevin continued to have episodes of respiratory distress of increasing severity and frequency. His clinical team and family agreed that the burden of further treatment outweighed any benefit. Therefore his advanced care plan was reviewed and amended with a plan to support end of life care at the hospice. Kevin was managed in accordance with an anticipatory symptom plan including the discontinuation of ventilator support and use of subcutaneous medications to minimise the need to give drugs by the enteral route. He died peacefully surrounded by his family.

After death, Kevin was moved to a specialist bedroom with cooling facilities, available in most hospices. Cold rooms can also be used by children who have died elsewhere e.g. in a hospital, as long as there is no restriction on moving the body. This enables family and friends to visit a patient after death. These facilities can also be made available in the home if families wish to take their infant/child/young person home as is common in some cultures.

If a child or young person dies in hospital then the hospital bereavement team will liaise closely with the family and support them in the hours and days after their child's death. They will help them with practical tasks including the timings of a post-mortem, organising to transfer the body to a funeral directors or a hospice, and advising them of the process of a Coroner's inquest if required by law. The bereavement team will arrange for the relevant documentation to be signed and instruct the family on how to register the death. After death, it is common practise for paediatric consultants to offer the family a bereavement visit to enable them to ask any questions and if necessary communicate or explain the results of post-mortem.

Syllabus Mapping

Palliative Care and Pain Management

- Know about end of life care and bereavement counselling and understand the opportunities for respite care, including the role of children's hopics

References

1. Children's palliative care definitions www.togetherforshortlives.org.uk/ last accessed 16/03/16

2. Guide to using the Advance Care Plan v1.6 http://cypacp.nhs.uk/ last accessed 16/03/16

3. Standards framework for children's palliative care (2015) www.togetherforshortlives.org.uk/ last accessed 16/03/16

4. www.childbereavementuk.org/ last accessed 23/2/16

5. www.winstonswish.org.uk/ last accessed 23/3/16

Further Reading

Brown, Erica and Warr, Brian (2007b) Supporting the Child and the Family in Paediatric Palliative Care. London: Jessica Kingsley Publishers

Goldman A., Hain R., and Liben S. (2012) Oxford Textbook of Palliative Care for Children. vol. Oxford textbooks in palliative medicine. Oxford: Oxford University Press

Pfund, Rita and Fowler-Kerry, Susan (2010a) Perspectives on Palliative Care for Children and Young People: a Global Discourse. New York: Radcliffe Publishing

Chapter 9: A major incident
Dr Simon Li

9

You are working in the emergency department. A major incident has been declared following a road traffic accident involving a school bus. A 12 year old boy arrives. His cervical spine is immobilised using head blocks. He is maintaining oxygen saturations of 94% with 10l/min oxygen by non-rebreathe facemask. "Snoring" sounds are audible from his nose and mouth. Heart rate is 148/minute, blood pressure 106/68 mmHg and capillary refill time 3 seconds centrally. He has an obvious open fracture of his left femur with continuing profuse haemorrhage.

Q1. Which of the following would you address first in his management?

A.   Excluding a cervical spine injury
B.   His oxygen saturations of 94%
C.   His reduced consciousness level
D.   The haemorrhage from his open fractured femur
E.   The snoring sounds that he is making

A 14 year old boy arrives on spinal board with his cervical spine immobilised.

Q2. Which one of the following clinical signs mandates an urgent CT scan?

A.   2 discreet episodes of vomiting
B.   4 cm firm haematoma overlying his occiput
C.   Bruising noted behind his left ear
D.   GCS of 14
E.   Laceration to his scalp

This is a list of traumatic injuries:

A.   Airway disruption
B.   Flail chest
C.   Lung collapse
D.   Massive haemothorax
E.   Open pneumothorax
F.   Pericardial tamponade
G.   Pulmonary contusion
H.   Rib fracture
I.   Simple pneumothorax
J.   Tension pneumothorax

For each of the following clinical scenarios choose the most likely diagnosis:

Q3a. A 10 year old boy complains of chest pain and difficulty in breathing. His oxygen saturations are 89% in 15l/min oxygen via a non-rebreathe trauma mask with a respiratory rate 54/minute. There is tracheal deviation to the left, with hyperresonant percussion and reduced air entry on the right hemithorax.

Q3b. A 15 year old girl is drowsy and has left sided chest wall bruising with fractures of her left 3rd, 4th and 5th ribs. She has stony dullness to percussion over her and reduced air entry in her left hemithorax.

Q3c. An 8 year old boy has bruising in the distribution of his seat belt. He is admitted overnight for observation and analgesia. The following day he complains of shortness of breath. A chest x-ray shows bilateral patchy consolidation.

Answers and Rationale

Q1.   D: The haemorrhage from his open fractured femur
Q2.   C: Bruising noted behind his left ear
Q3a.   J: Tension pneumothorax
Q3b.   D: Massive haemothorax
Q3c.   G: Pulmonary contusion

Trauma is not necessarily a domain within the curriculum that comes naturally to paediatricians. However, it is essential to be aware of how to initially manage trauma situations until further, more definitive, care can be arranged via a specialty team. As is the way within emergency paediatrics, using a structured approach allows timely detection and intervention of problems. This follows the path suggested by the Advanced Trauma Life Support (ATLS) algorithms which, although largely follows the usual "ABCDE" logic, has one notable revision. The ATLS paradigm is based on battlefield trauma in the military and advocates a <C>ABCDE approach (figure 9.1) which recognises the importance of catastrophic life-threatening haemorrhage which must be dealt with immediately. When control of catastrophic haemorrhage has been achieved, ABCDE is dealt with in the usual way.

Given this approach, the child in the first question requires haemorrhage control in the first instance given his open femoral fracture. In adults a closed fracture of the femur can lead to an estimated blood loss of 1000-1500ml which can be doubled in open fractures.

The question of the 14 year old who arrives on a spinal board is asking about the management of children who present with head injuries. This rather common presentation to the emergency department, has very clear management guidelines set out by National Institute for Health and Care Excellence (NICE) (1). This question focuses on the situation where CT head scans are indicated. Bruising is noted behind his left ear (Battle's sign) which is indicative of a base of skull fracture. Although rare, this type of fracture can cause meningeal tears resulting in leakage of cerebrospinal fluid and risk of meningitis. Because of the anatomical relationships to a variety of structures, damage to the skull base can also lead to haemorrhage as a result of damage to the internal carotid artery, or cranial nerve palsies secondary to cranial nerve damage. The other options in this question do not meet NICE criteria for an urgent CT brain.

The third question describes a number of respiratory signs which need to be pieced together. It is obvious that the 10 year old boy is in a great deal of respiratory distress and hypoxia is present despite generous oxygen supplementation via a non-rebreathe mask. The tracheal deviation to the left must mean that either there is left sided lung collapse (thus the trachea moves leftward to fill the void) or there is pathology within the right hemithorax great enough to push the trachea to the left. Percussion of the chest wall gives you the answer as there is hyperresonance over the right side of the chest meaning that there is excess air within the hemithorax i.e. a pneumothorax is present. This is confirmed on auscultation as there is reduced air entry on the left side. Simple pneumothorax would be insufficient to produce tracheal deviation and so the answer must be a tension pneumothorax. The emergency management of this is needle thoracocentesis followed by a definitive chest drain (2).

The pathology in the second case is across the entire left side of the child's chest and would fit with a diagnosis of a massive haemothorax. The findings on percussion of the chest wall makes use of the fact that striking a surface overlying a fluid filled cavity produces a deadened tone (dullness). Auscultation reveals reduced breath sounds as a result of the lack of aeration of the lung to hear any breathing. Management of this situation must be directed towards reducing the increased intrapleural pressure and associated lung collapse, and correcting the reduced blood volume and any associated haemodynamic instability. The haemothorax is removed from the pleural cavity with a chest drain. Rarely can the rapid evacuation of blood from within the chest cause haemodynamic collapse as a result of the intrapleural blood acting as a tamponade reducing the on-going blood loss from the intravascular space. Restoring the intravascular volume with a blood transfusion is also necessary (3).

The final question describes, other than for some whiplash, an apparently unscathed child involved in a road traffic accident. However it is not until the following day that symptoms become apparent with X-ray changes noted. These bilateral patchy changes are consistent with a diagnosis of pulmonary contusion. Its pathophysiology is worth noting and arises because a child's chest wall is very compliant which means that rib fractures do not often occur. This however is also a bad thing as paediatric chests do not dissipate force which means more of the impact force is applied directly to lung tissue. This force then causes blood and fluid to fill the alveoli, and a ventilation-perfusion mismatch which, in turn, leads to hypoxia. The management of this condition is good analgesia and supplemental oxygen as needed. Although pneumonia and acute respiratory distress syndrome are both documented complications of pulmonary contusion the outcome for children is excellent in comparison to adults who often develop long-term respiratory dysfunction.

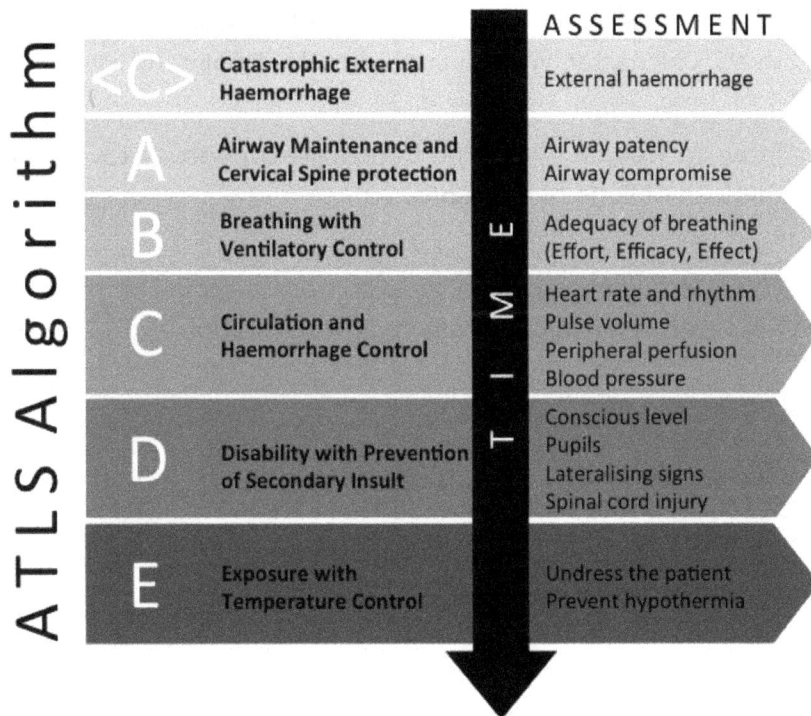

Figure 9.1: ATLS algorithm to the seriously injured child (Adapted from Schmidt et al.2009) (4)

Syllabus Mapping

Emergency Medicine (including accidents and poisoning)

- Know how to control acute blood loss until help arrives

- Know how to differentiate between life or limb threatening injuries and injuries that can be managed less urgently

- Know the principles of managing limb threatening injuries

- Know appropriate use of radiological investigations in trauma

- Know when to suspect and how to safely initiate management in head and spinal injury

References and Further Reading

1. National Institute for H, Care E. Head injury: triage, assessment, investigation and early management of head injury in children, young people and adults. London: NICE, 2014

2. Samuels M, Wieteska S, Advanced Life Support Group (Manchester England). Advanced paediatric life support: the practical approach. 5th ed. Chichester, West Sussex, UK: BMJ Books, 2011

3. American College of Surgeons. Committee on Trauma. Advanced trauma life support: ATLS ; student course manual. 9th ed. Chicago, IL.: American College of Surgeons, 2012

4. Schmidt OI, Gahr RH, Gosse A, et al. ATLS® and damage control in spine trauma. Modeling the two-hit hypothesis for evaluating strategies to prevent organ injury after shock/resuscitation. World Journal of Emergency Surgery 2009;4(1):1-11

Chapter 10: "Will she be asthmatic?"
Dr Arvind Shah, Dr Emily Isaacs and Dr Chris Dewhurst

10

Martha is a 4 year old child who attends her GP with what mum describes as a "wheeze". This is the fourth time she has attended the practice in the last 9 months with wheeze and on each occasion she had coryzal symptoms. She has been very breathless whilst playing but is alert and active in the clinic. Her temperature is 37.3⁰C, heart rate 120/minute and respiratory rate is 40 breaths per minute. She has mild intercostal recession with widespread wheeze on auscultation with transmitted noises. She has green nasal secretions.

Q1. Which of the following is the most appropriate management strategy?

A.   Inhaled beclomethasone
B.   Inhaled salbutamol
C.   Oral monteleukast
D.   Oral prednisolone
E.   Reassurance

Martha's mother wants to know if she is likely to develop asthma.

Q2. Which one of the following clinical features make it most likely that she will develop asthma?

A.   A history of allergic reaction to eggs
B.   A history of atopic dermatitis
C.   More than 6 wheezing episodes in 12 months
D.   Nocturnal Cough
E.   Wheezing unrelated to coryzal symptoms

Martha returns to the clinic 2 years later. She has had 2 admissions to hospital over the previous winter for 3 days requiring oxygen and nebulised therapy. She has been diagnosed as having asthma and commenced upon a salbutamol and steroid inhaler. Over the past 6 weeks she has been using her salbutamol inhaler almost every day and missed several days of school because of breathlessness.

Q3. What is the next step in her management?

A.   Ipratropium bromide inhaler
B.   Montelukast
C.   Oral steroids
D.   Oral theophylline
E.   Salmeterol (a long acting β_2 agonist)

Answers and Rationale

Q1.   B: Inhaled salbutamol
Q2.   B: A history of atopic dermatitis
Q3.   E: Salmeterol (a long acting β2 agonist)

It is important to confirm what is meant by wheezing when a parent volunteers this information. Wheeze can mean many different noises to parents, including transmitted noises, rattles, stridor and being breathless. True wheezing in pre-school children is however common, occurring in approximately a third of children less than 5 years old (1). Two distinct patterns of wheezing are seen in pre-school children (1):

Episodic viral wheeze

It is common for pre-school aged children to have around 6 respiratory tract infections per year. Airway inflammation and constriction of the bronchi, can result in wheeze and when these infections cause recurrent episodes of wheeze, this is known as episodic viral wheeze. In between the viral infections, the children are well. Infants who have had bronchiolitis in the first year of life are more likely to present in their pre-school years with episodic viral wheeze. The first question to ask when managing a child with episodic viral wheeze is whether they need treatment at all. The use of inhaled therapy to treat mild respiratory noises with minimal respiratory distress may be more problematic than the disease. Martha's breathlessness and marked wheeze would indicate the need for treatment, which would initially be with a bronchodilator. Montelukast treatment may be started to prevent winter-time wheezing episodes which result in hospital admission (2).

Multiple trigger wheeze

This is when a child wheezes not only with upper respiratory tract infections but also with other triggers such as exercise or exposure to allergens or smoke. Multiple trigger wheeze is part of the "atopic march" which proceeds through eczema, food allergies (particularly to cow's milk protein, nuts and egg), allergic rhinitis and asthma. In these children consideration of preventative treatment should be considered with either inhaled corticosteroids or leukotriene receptor antagonist (montelukast). Children with multiple trigger wheeze have a 50% chance of developing asthma (3). Those with no atopic personal or family history are more likely to "outgrow" their recurrent wheeze episodes as their airways enlarge and their immune system matures.

Parents often want to know if their pre-school child will go on to develop school age asthma. There are several predictive indices which will be useful when answering the question Martha's mother asks in question 2. These indices have a high negative predictive value and low positive predictive value. One such index is the asthma predictive index (API). It can be used for children aged 2 to 5 years with episodes of wheezing during the first 3 years of life (at least one diagnosed by a doctor), and predicts those more likely to develop asthma, if they have one major or at least two minor criteria from the list in (Table 33.1).

MAJOR CRITERIA	MINOR CRITERIA
• Parental history of asthma • Doctor diagnosed atopic dermatitis	• Blood eosinophils >4% • Wheezing unrelated to colds • Doctor diagnosed allergic rhinitis

Table 10.1: Asthma predictive index (4)

Asthma is a term to define children presenting with recurrent episodes of wheeze and breathlessness fluctuating over time and with treatment, often in the context of an atopic background (1, 4). The management of acute asthma is covered in chapter 28.

There are useful tools, such as the Asthma Control Test™ among others, which help in identifying patients with poorly controlled asthma, to guide management decisions (5,6).

Chronic management

SIGN advise treatment being commenced early to achieve symptom control and to step down management when control is good (6). The guidelines advise inhaler technique, adherence to medications and elimination of triggers to wheeze should be considered before increasing treatment. Checking inhaler technique is particularly relevant to children and every GP and paediatrician should know how to administer inhaled therapy effectively.

STEPS	Under 5 years	5-12 years
Mild, intermittent symptoms	• Short acting beta agonist	
1. Regular preventer therapy	• Regular (ICS) or Leukotriene receptor antagonist if steroid cannot be used	• Regular inhaled corticosteroid (ICS)
2. Initial add-on therapy	• Add leukotriene receptor antagonist (LTRA) to corticosteroid.	• Add long acting beta agonist (LABA) to ICS • If no LABA response, stop LABA, and continue to step 3 • If improvement with LABA but insufficient control, continue to step 3
3. Additional add-on therapies	• Increase ICS dose • Consider adding LTRA to therapy	
4. High dose therapies	Consider trials of: • Increasing ICS dose • Addition of a fourth drug e.g. slow release theophylline • Refer for specialist care	
Continuous or frequent use of oral steroids	• Use daily steroid tablet in lowest dose providing adequate control • Maintain medium-dose ICS • Consider other treatments to minimize use of steroid tablets • Refer for specialist care	

Table 10.2: SIGN management of chronic asthma (6)

SIGN (6) define "complete control" of asthma as:

No daytime symptoms

No night-time awakening due to asthma

No need for rescue medication

No asthma attacks

No limitations on activity including exercise (where relevant) normal lung function (in practical terms FEV1 and/or PEF>80% predicted or best)

Minimal side effects from medication

Complications of management

Inhaled corticosteroid therapy is considered safe and effective for children with asthma and improves their asthma control more than other treatment options. (6) There is debate as to whether inhaled corticosteroids affect growth, but long-term it is recognised that children with asthma who receive inhaled steroids reach average adult height. (6, 7) There was previous controversy surrounding use of LABAs in the under 12 age group, however, on a risk benefit basis they are considered safe in children, when ICS treatment is continued. (6, 8)

Syllabus Mapping

Respiratory Medicine with ENT

- Know how to assess and manage children with acute asthma and wheeze and plan long term management

- Understand the causes of chronic cough and appropriate investigations

- Understand the long term complications of medications used for asthma

References and Further Reading

1. Bush A, Grigg J, Saglani S. Managing wheeze in preschool children. BMJ. 2014 Feb 4;348:g15

2. Yunginger JW, Reed CE, O'Connell EJ, Melton III LJ, O'Fallon WM, Silverstein MD. A community-based study of the epidemiology of asthma: incidence rates, 1964–1983. American Review of Respiratory Disease. 1992 Oct;146(4):888-94

3. Rhodes HL, Thomas P, Sporik R, Holgate ST, Cogswell JJ. A birth cohort study of subjects at risk of atopy: twenty-two–year follow-up of wheeze and atopic status. American journal of respiratory and critical care medicine. 2002 Jan 15;165(2):176-80

4. Castro-Rodríguez JA, Holberg CJ, Wright AL, Martinez FD. A clinical index to define risk of asthma in young children with recurrent wheezing. American journal of respiratory and critical care medicine. 2000 Oct 1;162(4):1403-6

5. Asthma Control Test™ at http://www.asthma.com/additional-resources/asthma-control-test.html Published: 2002. Last accessed:06/04/2016

6. SIGN 153 British guideline on the management of asthma. http://www.sign.ac.uk/pdf/SIGN153.pdf, Last accessed 15/01/2017

7. Agertoft L, Pedersen S. Effect of long-term treatment with inhaled budesonide on adult height in children with asthma. N Engl J Med. 2000 Oct 12;343(15):1064-9

8. US Food and Drug Administration. FDA Drug Safety Communication: New safety requirements for long-acting inhaled asthma medications called Long-Acting Beta-Agonists (LABA). Human Department of Health and Human services. Feb 18, 2010. 1-4

Chapter 11: A floppy newborn
Dr Victoria McKay

You are called to the postnatal ward to see a female infant born 4 hours ago at term weighing of 3.0 kg (9th-25th centile). She is the second child to a 40 year old healthy mother and her partner. There is no significant family history, the couple have had no previous miscarriages and their eldest daughter is 2 years old, fit and healthy. During pregnancy the couple declined all antenatal serum screening tests. The midwife is concerned that the baby may be dysmorphic and the parents are now very anxious.

On examination she is hypotonic and sleepy but taking formula milk slowly by bottle. She has brachycephaly with a flat occiput and wrinkled skin on the back of her neck. Her tongue is protruding; she has epicanthic folds and up-slanting palpebral fissures. You hear a loud murmur when you auscultate her chest but she is pink and well perfused. You think she may have some spots on her iris and she appears to have a convergent strabismus (squint).

Q1. What clinical investigation would be best to arrange next?

A. Auditory brainstem response (ABR) hearing test
B. Echocardiogram
C. Ophthalmological examination
D. Renal ultrasound scan
E. Thyroid function tests

Q2. Which genetic test would be best to confirm the diagnosis?

A. DNA sequencing
B. Flow cytometry
C. Karyotype
D. Microarray (competitive genomic hybridisation array (CGHarray))
E. Rapid aneuploidy screen (quantitative fluorescence polymerise chain reaction)

Q3. What is the most likely genetic mechanism to have caused this condition?

A. Maternal meiotic non-disjunction
B. Mosaicism
C. Point mutation
D. Reciprocal translocation
E. Robertsonian translocation

Answers and Rationale

Q1. **B: Echocardiogram**
Q2. **E: Rapid aneuploidy screen (quantitative fluorescence polymerise chain reaction**
Q3. **A: Maternal meiotic non-disjunction**

This baby has Down syndrome, also known as trisomy 21. Down syndrome is caused by having 3 copies (trisomy) of chromosome 21 instead of the normal 2 copies (disomy). It is important that you recognise when dysmorphic features are present in a neonate and have an understanding of any potential associated conditions the baby may have. In newborns with DS the immediate health issues are confirming the cardiac anatomy and ensuring there is no bowel obstruction, most commonly secondary to duodenal atresia.

Down Syndrome is one of the 3 common trisomies and can be diagnosed within 24-48 hours using a rapid aneuploidy screen (RAS). RAS will confirm or exclude a diagnosis of Down syndrome where there are concerning clinical features. If Down syndrome is confirmed, the mechanism causing the trisomy 21 can subsequently be defined with a full karyotype. The full karyotype will take approximately 2 weeks and in 95% of cases will show that the cause of the trisomy 21 is maternal meiotic non-disjunction, which is related to increased maternal age.

Neonates with Down syndrome are often markedly hypotonic and may be difficult to wake for feeds (1). The facial features of epicanthic folds (small folds of skin across the medial aspects of the eyes), up-slanting palpebral fissures (where a line drawn from the medial to lateral aspects of the eye points upwards), small ears, protruding tongue and excess nuchal skin, may prompt clinical suspicion of the diagnosis. However these features may be more difficult to determine in certain babies, depending on their ethnic background or in premature babies.

40% of patients with Down syndrome have congenital heart disease (CHD), most commonly AVSD but other septal and valvular defects are also common (2). All neonates with confirmed Down syndrome should have an echocardiogram in the postnatal period with cardiology follow-up if CHD is detected. Routine neonatal screening should also be completed, including audiology screening and the newborn blood spot. Screening is particularly important for babies with Down syndrome as there is an increased incidence of conductive and sensorineural hearing loss and hypothyroidism (2). You should be familiar with your local pathways for children newly diagnosed with Down syndrome and this may involve arranging other referrals before discharge, for example renal ultrasound scans and community paediatric follow-up. Ophthalmological review in the first few months of life is appropriate, but hypo-pigmented spots on the iris (Brushfield spots) and the appearance of pseudostrabismus created by epicanthic folds do not cause visual problems.

It is important that you involve a senior colleague when you think the clinical features in a neonate may suggest Down syndrome, so that the diagnosis can be confirmed and parents informed in a timely and sensitive manner. When discussing the diagnosis it is important to maintain a balance between being realistic about the future and not focussing heavily on potential negative aspects of the condition.

Parents are likely to need some degree of support in the time immediately following diagnosis and could be directed to the national support group, the Down Syndrome Association (3).

In the antenatal period suspicion of Down syndrome may be raised by the finding of typical structural anomalies such as CHD or duodenal atresia or by serum screening results. Maternal serum screening uses a combination of serum markers to give a likelihood of Down syndrome. The markers measured in the mother's blood include alpha-fetoprotein (AFP), unconjugated oestriol (uE3), inhibin A and human chorionic gonadotropin (HCG). The results of these tests are combined with maternal age to give an overall risk in the fetus (4). It is important that parents are aware that this test gives only a probability of having a baby with Down syndrome and that a low risk does not mean that there is zero chance. Some couples will choose not to have any serum screening as it would not alter the decisions they would make regarding continuing with a pregnancy. Some couples would opt for an invasive procedure such as a chorionic villous biopsy or amniocentesis if they felt their risk was high enough. Some couples would choose to end a pregnancy if Down syndrome was confirmed.

Genetic Diagnosis

RAS is a way of quickly counting the number of copies of chromosomes 13, 18, 21 and the sex chromosomes. It is therefore a useful and rapid test to look for aneuploidies (abnormalities in the number of chromosomes). It should be the first test requested if there is clinical suspicion of these conditions and will usually provide a result in 24-48 hours. RAS is often now performed using a method known as QF-PCR, but can also be performed using fluorescence in situ hybridisation (FISH) (5).

If a diagnosis of trisomy 21 is found on RAS, the lab will then proceed to a full karyotype, where all of the chromosomes are visualised. This is a much longer process, taking approximately 2 weeks to complete, but has the advantage of being able to determine how the trisomy 21 was caused. In approximately 95% of cases, trisomy 21 is caused by maternal meiotic non-disjunction (1). This means that two copies of chromosome 21 did not separate in maternal meiosis. Non-disjunction is more likely to occur as women age and this is reflected in the incidence of DS of 1 in 1500 with a maternal age of 20 at delivery, compared to an incidence of 1 in 100 with a maternal age of 40. After having one baby with Down syndrome secondary to non-disjunction, the chance of a second baby would be age-related and not significantly higher than for other mothers of the same age.

Less commonly, trisomy 21 can be caused by other mechanisms, including Robertsonian translocations in 4% and mosaicism in 1% (1). Mosaicism occurs when the trisomy 21 is not present in every cell in the body and can cause variable clinical features. A Robertsonian translocation occurs when two chromosomes lose their short arms and their long arms subsequently stick together. If this includes chromosome 21 then the outcome could be a baby with Down syndrome or recurrent miscarriages. If a full karyotype shows that trisomy 21 was caused by any mechanism other than non-disjunction, the family should be referred to clinical genetics for further counselling.

There are many new genetic technologies in use to facilitate non-invasive diagnoses in pregnancies deemed to be at high risk of Down syndrome. This includes sequencing cell-free DNA (cfDNA) detected in maternal plasma to determine how many copies of chromosome 21 are present (6). This has huge potential for application to non-invasive prenatal testing in the future.

Other Common Aneuploidies

Other aneuploidies may be suspected clinically in either the antenatal or neonatal period. Patau syndrome (trisomy 13) presents with multiple, complex congenital anomalies, including holoprosencephaly (failure of the brain to divide into two separate hemispheres), orofacial clefts and polydactyly . Edward syndrome (trisomy 18) presents with prenatal growth deficiency, over-riding fingers and CHD. These trisomies are usually associated with significantly shortened life span. Clinical genetics departments may be available to provide input where a trisomy is suspected or diagnosed.

Turner syndrome and Klinefelter syndrome are known as sex chromosome aneuploidies, as they are due to a change in the number of sex chromosomes. Girls with Turner syndrome may present with aortic arch abnormalities, webbing of the neck and pedal lymphoedema. They can however remain asymptomatic, even into adulthood. They have a karyotype of 45, X and this is often associated with other minor X-chromosome abnormalities (7). Boys with Klinefelter syndrome have a karyotype of 47, XXY and are often not diagnosed until later in childhood or even in adult life. They may have tall stature, behavioural problems or present with infertility. They too can however remain asymptomatic. All the aneuploidies can be diagnosed quickly with RAS and confirmed with a full karyotype.

Syllabus Mapping

Genetics and Dysmorphology

- Understand patterns of disease inheritance and be able to construct a family tree and interpret patterns of inheritance

- Know about the features of common chromosome disorders e.g. Down, Turner and Fragile X syndromes

- Know the basis of genetic screening and diagnosis, the common conditions for which they are used and the ethical dilemmas they pose

- Know about environmental factors which may affect pre-natal development e.g. maternal health, alcohol and drugs

References and Further Reading

1. Mueller RF and Young ID. Emery's Elements of Medical Genetics. London, UK; Churchill Livingston 2001:249-66

2. Hunter AGW. Down Syndrome. In: Cassidy SB and Allanson JE Eds. Management of Genetic Syndromes. Hoboken, New Jersey: John Wiley & Sons, Inc. 2010:309-35

3. http://www.downs-syndrome.org.uk/for-new-parents/ . Last accessed December 2015

4. Kliegman RM, Marcdante KJ, Jenson HB et al. Nelson Essentials of Paediatrics. Philadelphia, USA: Elsevier Saunders 2006:231-41

5. http://www.geneticseducation.nhs.uk/laboratory-process-and-testing-techniques/qf-pcr Last accessed December 2015

6. Nicolaides KH, Wright D, Poon LC, Syngelaki A, Gil MM. First-trimester contingent screening for trisomy 21 by biomarkers and maternal blood cell-free DNA testing. Ultrasound in Obstetrics & Gynecology. 2013 Jul 1;42(1):41-50

7. Davenport ML. Turner Syndrome. In: Cassidy SB and Allanson JE Eds. Management of Genetic Syndromes. Hoboken, New Jersey: John Wiley & Sons, Inc. 2010:847-69

Chapter 12: The baby with a lump, bump and bruise
Dr Chris Dewhurst

12

David is an 8 day old baby who is brought to the emergency department by his 19 year old mother. She is concerned about a lump that she has felt on his collarbone. He was born at term weighing 4.6 kg following a vacuum extraction. He sleeps for 3 hours at a time and wakes to take his artificial milk feeds.

On examination he is clean, asleep and appears well. His weight and head circumference are both on the 25th centile. He has generalised bruising to the crown of his head and circular bruising to both sides of his chest. There is a lump on his left clavicle. His frenulum is intact. On examining his nappy area there is severe ammoniacal dermatitis (erythematous patches and scaling, the skin folds are spared). You dilate his pupils and on direct ophthalmoscopy see retinal haemorrhages. There are no other obvious injuries. Examination of his chest, heart and abdomen is normal.

You arrange an x-ray of his clavicle that demonstrates a fracture.

Q1. Which one of the following findings in David is most suggestive of non-accidental injury?

A.	Bruising to the crown
B.	Fractured clavicle
C.	Oval shaped bruising to both sides of the chest
D.	Retinal haemorrhages
E.	Severe ammoniacal dermatitis

Q2. What is the most important next investigation for David?

A.	25-hydroxyvitamin D serum levels
B.	Calcium and phosphate serum levels
C.	Coagulation Screen
D.	CT head scan
E.	Skeletal Survey

Q3. Who should you contact next?

A.	General Practitioner
B.	Health Visitor
C.	Police
D.	Social care service
E.	The child's father

Answers and Rationale

Q1.   C: Oval shaped bruising to both sides of the chest
Q2.   D: CT head scan
Q3.   D: Social care service

Protecting children from intentional harm is the duty of every paediatrician. Cases such as the one described above can often be difficult to deal with and cause great anxiety and uncertainty for the attending doctor. However, the investigation and management of cases where children may be abused should be approached with the same systematic and rigorous manner as you would for any other life threatening illness (as suggested by Lord Laming in the Victoria Climbie enquiry) (1). As always, this starts with a history, examination and further investigations if required.

When faced with a safeguarding question, the age of the patient and history are key to determining the correct answer. David is an 8 day old baby and is presenting with several findings, many of which may be a sign of non-accidental injury in older children but at this age may be related to his birth. For example, clavicular fractures are the most common fracture following birth, occurring in up to 3% of deliveries (2). The fracture may not be apparent at birth and remain asymptomatic. The presence of a "lump" indicates callous formation meaning that the fractures occurred at least 7 days earlier, i.e. around the time of his delivery. If however a fractured clavicle was seen in a baby more than a month of age this would be more likely related to non-accidental injury than an accident (3).

Whilst bruising is the commonest injury in children who have been physically abused, children also sustain bruises from every day play activities and accidents (4). When determining the potential cause of bruising, the age of the child is absolutely critical. Bruising is strongly related to mobility and accidental bruising is uncommon in babies who are not yet crawling and therefore have no independent mobility. However bruising following delivery occurs relatively commonly and the description of bruising to the crown in this case is due to a chignon following vacuum extraction. The circular bruising on the chest is most likely fingertip bruising. Grabbing and/or squeezing causes this, leaving oval shaped bruises. Not all of the fingers may leave a bruise due uneven pressure being applied. This type of bruising is highly suggestive of non-accidental injury and would be uncommon to see as a result of the birth process.

Retinal haemorrhages are strongly associated with abusive head trauma. In the under 3's the odds ratio for abusive head trauma when retinal haemorrhages are found is 15.3 (5). However, retinal haemorrhages occur in approximately 1 in 4 neonates following spontaneous vaginal delivery and are strongly associated with vacuum extraction. Follow up studies have demonstrated that retinal haemorrhages following birth usually resolve within 2 weeks but may still be present up to 42 days after birth (5). Therefore, if seen at 8 days of life, isolated retinal haemorrhages may relate to the birth process rather than abusive head trauma. Given the fingertip bruising in this case however, the retinal haemorrhages may in fact be related to an abusive head injury.

Severe ammoniacal dermatitis can occur when there is infrequent nappy changing, which in itself may be a sign of neglect. Parental education may be all that is required but other concerning features in the history or examination may warrant further investigation.

Investigations in potential non-accidental injury cases include those looking for occult injuries (e.g. skeletal surveys for fractures, CT scan of the head for intracranial bleeds and/or abdominal imaging for organ injury) and those investigating for potential medical causes for observed injuries (e.g. platelets and clotting studies in bruising, vitamin D and bone profile in fractures etc.). In this case (Table 12.1), the CT scan is more important to arrange than the skeletal survey as this may demonstrate haemorrhage which needs immediate neurosurgical intervention.

Skeletal surveys are indicated in all children under 2 years who are suspected of being physically abused and in older children when there are fractures suggestive of abuse (6). Recent guidance on which fractures are more suggestive of abuse has been produced highlighting that up to 56% of all fractures in children under one year of age were due to abuse (7). Repeating the skeletal survey after 2 weeks may reveal previously undiagnosed fractures and can help in the dating of the fracture.

Bruising	Fractures
Coagulation screen Prothrombin time Activated partial thromboplastin time Thrombin Time Fibrinogen	**Skeletal survey:** All children < 2 year where physical abuse is suspected Older children dependant on history, examination and fracture type
Full blood count and film	**CT head scan:** All children < 1 year where physical abuse is suspected Older children dependant on history and examination
Factor VIIIc	**Bone biochemistry:**
Von Willebrand factor	Calcium and phosphate Alkaline phosphatase Serum 25-hydroxyvitamin D Parathyroid hormone

Table 12.1: First line investigations in suspected physical abuse. Other investigations may be necessary depending on clinical findings and results of first line investigations adapted from (6, 7)

Safeguarding children involves working in partnership with the family and professionals from other agencies. The information known to you as the attending paediatrician may only reflect a small part of the family's life. There may be many different professionals involved in supporting the family including health visitors, general practitioners, family support workers, social workers, drug and alcohol workers, youth offending teams, housing agencies etc. Each of these professionals may have small pieces of information that when put together build a picture of the family's life. It is the responsibility of the paediatrician to recognise and report when abuse may be occurring and to assist statutory agencies (Police, Social services and the NSPCC) in the investigation of potential abuse. The first agency to contact is often the local social care service as they may have information about the family from other agencies and be aware if the child is on a child protection plan.

Syllabus Mapping

Neonatology

*   Be able to recognise and assess birth injury with appropriate referral

Safeguarding

*   Know the presentations of physical, emotional and sexual abuse, neglect and fabricated and induced illness

*   Know what steps should be taken when child abuse is suspected

References

1. Laming Report (2003) The Victoria Climbié Inquiry. Report of an inquiry by Lord Laming. HMSO, London

2. Joseph PR, Rosenfeld W. Clavicular fractures in neonates. Archives of Pediatrics & Adolescent Medicine 1990 Feb 1;144(2):165.

3. Pandya NK, Baldwin K, Wolfgruber H, Christian CW, Drummond DS, Hosalkar HS. Child abuse and orthopaedic injury patterns: analysis at a level I pediatric trauma center. Journal of Pediatric Orthopaedics 009;29(6):618-625

4. Maguire S, Mann M. Systematic reviews of bruising in relation to child abuse—what have we learnt: an overview of review updates. Evidence Based Child Health: A Cochrane Review Journal. 2013;8:255–263

5. Maguire SA, Watts PO, Shaw AD, Holden S, Taylor RH, Watkins WJ, Mann MK, Tempest V, Kemp AM. Retinal haemorrhages and related findings in abusive and non-abusive head trauma: A systematic review Eye 2013; 27:28-36

6. Royal College of Paediatrics and Child Health. Child protection companion - 2nd edition. 2013

7. Borg K, Hodes D. Guidelines for skeletal survey in young children with fractures. Archives of disease in childhood-Education & practice edition. 2015 Jan 14:edpract-2014

Further Reading

Cardiff Child Protection Systematic Reviews – CORE INFO. http://www.core-info.cardiff.ac.uk/reviews/fractures/which-fractures-are-indicative-of-abuse. (Last accessed 5th February 2016)

Chapter 13: The 'jumpy' baby
Dr Jane Elizabeth Valente and Dr Jane Hassell

Kiran is a 3 week old boy who is brought to the emergency department by his mother with a history of abnormal 'jumpy' movements of the right arm that occurred for the first time this morning. For the past 2 days he has been sleepier than normal and he has not been breast feeding as well as usual. He was born at term following a normal vaginal delivery weighing 3.7 kg and was discharged home at 6 hours.

On examination he is lying in his mother's arms looking lethargic. His heart rate is 120/minute, blood pressure 80/50mmHg with a capillary refill time of less than 2 seconds centrally. He is floppy but there are no focal neurological signs. His fontanelle is normal. He has a temperature of 36°C and his blood sugar is 3.7 mmol/l.

Q1. Which one of the following investigations is the most important?

A.   C-reactive protein
B.   Electroencephalogram (EEG)
C.   Lumbar puncture
D.   Serum Calcium
E.   Urine microscopy and culture

Q2. Which one of the following would be your first line management for this infant?

A.   Amoxicillin and Gentamicin
B.   Cefotaxime, Amoxicillin and Acyclovir
C.   Glucose bolus
D.   Normal saline bolus
E.   Pyridoxine bolus

Q3. What is the most likely diagnosis?

A.   Benign neonatal seizures
B.   Hypoglycaemia
C.   Infantile spasms
D.   Meningoencephalitis
E.   Septicaemia

Answers and Rationale

Q1.   **C: Lumbar puncture**
Q2.   **B: Cefotaxime, Amoxicillin and Acyclovir**
Q3.   **D: Meningoencephalitis**

All healthcare professionals, but particularly those dealing directly with neonates such as GP's, midwives and pediatricians, must be able to recognise the unwell neonate. Kiran has presented with nonspecific signs and a possible history of focal fitting. First, determine if the history of the jerky right arm does indeed reflect abnormal movements. Parents will often video any abnormal movements on smartphones or cameras and this can be useful in helping to determine normal baby movements from abnormal seizure activity. However, not all abnormal movements in babies are seizures and the clinical interpretation of seizure from non-seizure activity can be very difficult. In Kiran's case there are features indicating that he is unwell making it more likely that the jerky arm movements do indeed represent focal seizure activity. These features are:

- lethargy
- poor feeding
- hypothermia

There are multiple causes of seizures in this age group (see Table 13.1). Often the underlying cause can be determined from the history, including the pregnancy, family history, and physical examination. If the cause of seizures is unclear from the history and examination the following tests are useful in determining the underlying cause (1):

- Blood glucose, calcium, magnesium, urea, electrolytes and acid-base status
- Full blood count and film
- CSF analysis
- Blood, CSF and urine cultures
- Cranial ultrasound scan

Further investigations performed depend upon the clinical presentation and the results of the initial evaluations include blood ammonia, lactate, uric acid, liver enzymes, biotinidase levels, blood and urine amino acids, urine organic acids, urine reducing substances, torch screen, MRI brain, genetic testing and EEG.

Sepsis should be your first consideration with an unwell neonate that has had a seizure. Both neonatal bacterial meningitis and, more rarely, neonatal encephalitis must be considered. Both diagnoses are supported in Kiran's case by the presence of lethargy. Other symptoms indicative of a diagnosis of neonatal meningitis may include jitteriness, vomiting, diarrhoea, abdominal distension, dyspnoea, cyanosis, hyperthermia, irritability, bulging fontanelle and, more rarely, sunset eyes. It must be remembered that neonates presenting with meningitis or encephalitis can present in a variety of non-specific signs and symptoms with no history of fitting. The most likely bacterial causes of meningitis in this case are group B streptococcus (GBS), Escherichia coli and Listeria monocytogenes.

Neonatal encephalitis is much rarer than bacterial meningitis and is most commonly caused by the maternal vertical transmission of herpes simplex virus. A history of maternal genital herpes and a vaginal delivery increases the risk of neonatal herpes encephalitis. It presents in a similar way to bacterial meningitis and is diagnosed by the positive cerebrospinal fluid (CSF) viral culture of herpes simplex virus (HSV). Most cases also display an abnormal EEG. Antiviral drug therapy with acyclovir is the most common treatment (2).

If infants with neonatal meningitis or encephalitis are not treated promptly the results can be catastrophic with death or long term disability being the consequence (3). In this case neonatal bacterial meningitis is the most likely diagnosis but the rarer diagnosis of neonatal encephalitis must also be treated until a diagnosis can been made. The diagnosis of neonatal bacterial meningitis is made by cerebrospinal fluid (CSF) examination via a lumbar puncture (LP). A positive result is indicated by one or more of the following: isolation of a bacterium, an increased white blood cell count, a raised protein level and a decreased glucose concentration.

An infant in a poor clinical condition should be treated immediately with antibiotics and antivirals as delaying treatment can have disastrous consequences (even if this means delaying the lumbar puncture). A combination of broad spectrum antibiotics including cover for listeria (such as ampicillin) and anti-viral medication (such as acyclovir) is important until CSF cultures are available (4). Kiran is not in shock as he has normal capillary refill and normal blood pressure. Thus, while he will require fluid treatment if his fluid intake is reduced, he does not require a bolus of normal saline at this stage. Hypoglycemia, hypocalcaemia, hyponatraemia, hypernatraemia and hypomagnesaemia can present with non-specific signs, symptoms and/or seizures so blood should be taken for a glucose and electrolyte/calcium/magnesium measurements when an intravenous cannula is inserted. Infantile spasms are a specific type of seizure disorder which would not normally be present, as in this case, with a focal seizure. They usually present with a sudden tonic contraction of the trunk and limb muscles lasting on average 5-10 seconds with spasms often happening in quick succession. West's syndrome usually occurs between 4 and 8 months rather than in the neonatal period and consists of infantile spasms, developmental regression and hypsarrythmia on the EEG. Growth delay and signs specific to the aetiology, most commonly tuberous sclerosis may be noted when this condition presents at a later age. Hypsarrhythmia is characteristically seen on the EEG. Treatment is usually with corticosteroids or newer drugs such as vigabatrin and in general the intellectual prognosis is poor.

Diagnosis	Tests to establish diagnosis
Infections Septicaemia/Meningitis/Encephalitis/Toxoplasmosis/Cytomegalovirus	Blood cultures/CSF
Metabolic disorders Hypoglycaemia/Hyponatraemia/Hypernatraemia/Hypocalcaemia/hypomagnasaemia/Inborn errors of metabolism	Blood glucose/Electrolytes/Magnesium/Calcium/Metabolic screen (urine and plasma)
Intracranial Haemorrhage	Head ultrasound scan
Congenital Brain Malformations	CT/MRI brain scan
Infantile spasms	EEG
Benign neonatal seizures	EEG
Pyridoxine deficiency	Therapeutic trial of pyridoxine

Table 13.1: Differential diagnosis of abnormal movements/seizures in a neonate

Syllabus Mapping

Neonatology

- Be able to recognise and initiate the management of common disorders in the newborn including sepsis

- Be aware of the occurrence and clinical features of maternal to fetal transmission of infection

- Know the presentations of neonatal seizures and recognise abnormal neurological features e.g. the floppy baby

Neurology

- Know the likely causes and management of meningitis/encephalitis and altered consciousness

- Know the causes and presentation of seizure disorders, their differential diagnosis, the principles of management and when to refer

References and Further Reading

1. Lecture Notes. Chapter 23 Investigation of seizures in infant. Richard Appleton and Ailsa McLellan. Available at https://www.epilepsysociety.org.uk/sites/default/files/attachments/Chapter23McLellan2015.pdf

2. Le Doare K. Min consultation: Managing neonatal and childhood herpes encephalitis. Arch Dis Child Educ Pract Ed pii: edpract-2014-306321. 15

3. Wiswell TE, Baumgart S, Gannon CM, Spitzer AR. No lumbar puncture in the evaluation for early neonatal sepsis: will meningitis be missed? Pediatrics 1995; 95:803

4. Kessler SL, Dajani AS. Listeria meningitis in infants and children. The Pediatric infectious disease journal. 1990 Jan 1;9(1):61-2

Chapter 14: A breathless baby
Dr Poothirikovil Venugopalan

Tom is a 2 month old baby boy who is brought to the children's emergency department by his parents with a history of poor feeding and shortness of breath for the past 2 days.

He was born at full term by normal delivery weighing 3.7 kg (75th centile). He was discharged home at 4 hours of age at parental request. He remained well but at his routine 6 week review his GP noted that his weight of 4.0 kg was now on the 25th centile and he had a cardiac murmur. His GP referred him to the paediatric outpatient clinic which is scheduled for 1 months' time.

On examination he is pink, saturating 95% in air with a respiratory rate 70/minute, heart rate 150/minute and temperature 37°C. Capillary refill is 2 seconds centrally and peripherally. He has a depressed nasal bridge, upward slanting palpebral fissures and bilateral simian creases. He is hypotonic with normal deep tendon reflexes.

He has chest recession with clear lung fields on auscultation. His heart sounds are normal with, a grade 3/6 pansystolic murmur audible loudest over the lower left sternal border that conducts all over the chest. His abdomen is soft with a palpable liver of 4 cm.

Q1. What is the single most important examination to now perform?

A.   Auscultate the carotid arteries
B.   Examine the iris
C.   Inspect the palate
D.   Palpate femoral pulses
E.   Palpate for splenomegaly

Q2. What would be the most likely diagnosis in this baby?

A.   Innocent heart murmur
B.   Large atrial septal defect
C.   Large ventricular septal defect
D.   Severe aortic stenosis
E.   Small ventricular septal defect

Q3. Which one of the following specialists do you refer this child to next?

A.   Anaesthetist to admit to PICU
B.   Cardiologist to manage medically
C.   Cardiothoracic surgeons for urgent surgical repair
D.   Dietician to optimise nutrition
E.   Geneticist for genetic testing

Answers and Rationale

Q1. D: Palpate femoral pulses
Q2. C: Large ventricular septal defect
Q3. B: Cardiologist to manage medically

To answer this question we need to revisit our basic physical examination skills. A cardiovascular examination is not complete by just describing the heart murmur. Clues to the underlying heart defect will be identified form the general physical examination which may identify signs of heart failure or dysmorphic features which may increase your suspicion of the underlying defect (1). It is of paramount importance to palpate the femoral pulses and look for brachio-femoral or radio-femoral delay to identify the presence of a co-existing coarctation of the aorta. In this case the dysmorphic features are suggestive of a baby with Down syndrome. Children with Down syndrome have a high incidence of congenital heart defects (40%). The most common defect is an atrioventricular septal defect (20%), with ventricular septal defects (<10%), and atrial septal defects (10%) also being relatively common (2). In this case the clinical features of normal heart sounds with a grade 3/6 pansystolic cardiac murmur best heard over the lower left sternal border, and widely conducted are highly suggestive of a ventricular septal defect. It is worth noting that an atrioventricular septal defect, with valve regurgitation can also present with a similar murmur (Table 14.1). Confirmation of the diagnosis requires further investigations including a chest x-ray, ECG and echocardiogram.

Tom's normal oxygen saturation of 95% also helps to confirm that this is a left to right shunt lesion. The history given by the parents is helpful in that the symptoms were noticed at the 6-week check-up, as is often the case with ventricular septal defects (the pulmonary vascular resistance is high in the newborn period and this limits the volume of the left to right shunt during the first few weeks of life).

The general physical examination confirms poor weight gain, tachypnoea and clear lung fields which suggest heart failure. Heart failure is a feature of a large rather than a small ventricular septal defect. Because the baby is in heart failure the initial management would include stabilisation and initiation of diuretics under guidance of the cardiologist. Further investigations would include blood chemistry and karyotype. It is likely that Tom will need an early surgical repair of the heart defect, but in the absence of a coarctation or other complex congenital cardiac malformations, surgical repair can be scheduled in the subsequent 3-4 months.

Heart Murmurs: The majority of heart murmurs heard in children are benign or innocent cardiac murmurs. These are usually short systolic murmurs grade 2/6, loudest over the lower left sternal border and the child is otherwise well. Causes of pathological murmurs are described in (Table 14.1).

Additional Information: The majority of heart defects are multifactorial in origin with an overall prevalence of 8-10/1000 live births. However there are specific chromosomal associations as well as genetic syndromes which have a predisposition to certain types of congenital heart defects (4). Recognised associations include supravalvular aortic stenosis with William's syndrome, dysplastic pulmonary valve with Noonan syndrome, Truncus arteriosus and Tetralogy of Fallot with 22 q deletion and atrial septal defects with Holt-Oram syndrome. Maternal alcohol abuse as well as medications like phenytoin during pregnancy can also lead to heart defects in the baby. Gestational diabetes during pregnancy is associated with hypertrophic cardiomyopathy in the neonatal eriod, which usually resolves spontaneously.

The congenital heart diseases may present with cyanosis, heart failure or a combination of both. Ventricular septal defect, atrioventricular septal defect and patent ductus arteriosus manifest symptoms of heart failure. Tetralogy of Fallot, Transposition of great arteries and total anomalous pulmonary venous drainage present generally with cyanosis or low oxygen saturations (Table 14.2). Pulmonary stenosis, aortic stenosis and atrial septal defect present as asymptomatic murmurs except when severe. Coarctation of the aorta if severe, can present in the newborn period with heart failure or collapse, while less severe coarctation may go undetected in infancy and present later with upper limb hypertension.

Site of murmur	Systolic	Diastolic	Continuous
Cardiac apex	Mitral regurgitation	Mitral stenosis	
Lower left sternal border	Ventricular septal defect Tricuspid regurgitation Common atrioventricular valve with regurgitation		
Upper left sternal border	Pulmonary stenosis Patent ductus arteriosus Atrial septal defect Aortic stenosis	Pulmonary regurgitation Aortic regurgitation	Patent ductus arteriosus
Neck/aortic area	Aortic stenosis		Venous hum
Back	Coarctation of the aorta Pulmonary stenosis		Coarctation of the aorta AVmalformations

Table 14.1: Cardiac murmurs with different congenital heart defects

The presence of a congenital heart defect renders the heart and great vessels prone to bacterial growths that can present with systemic features of infection and worsening cardiac symptoms secondary to the damage produced by these bacterial growths (vegetations). Rarely fungi and viruses can also cause endocarditis. While evaluating children with congenital heart defects one needs to look for pointers to endocarditis like prolonged fever, splinter haemorrhages, Osler nodes, clubbing, splenomegaly and microscopic haematuria. Prompt investigations including repeated blood cultures should be obtained prior to commencing antibiotics. Maintaining good dental hygiene by regular brushing twice a day, prompt attention to dental caries, and avoiding tattoos and piercings will reduce the risk of endocarditis. All carers and older children with congenital heart defects should be counselled on these measures and also informed of the symptoms of endocarditis, especially prolonged fever (to facilitate early diagnosis). Regular antibiotic prophylaxis following dental procedures has not been shown to reduce the incidence of subsequent endocarditis, moreover such a practice may favour antibiotic resistant bacteria in the oral cavity and is now not recommended (3).

Central	Peripheral
Causes	**Causes**
Congenital heart diseases	Sluggish circulation
Pulmonary diseases	Heart failure
Abnormal haemoglobins	Shock
(methemoglobin/sulfhemoglobin)	Exposure to cold temperatures
	Arterial obstruction (Raynaud)
	Venous obstruction (Deep vein thrombosis)
Clinical features	
Affects whole body	
Skin and mucosa blue	**Clinical features**
Pulse oximetry abnormal	Often localised to the peripheries
	Skin may be blue but mucosa pink
	Pulse oximetry generally normal

Table 14.2: Central and peripheral cyanosis

Syllabus Mapping

Cardiology

- Know the clinical features of common congenital heart conditions and understand the principles of management

- Know the common causes of cyanosis and how to assess these

- Know the causes of murmurs palpitations, syncope and chest pain understand the principles of management and when to refer

- Know the causes and clinical features of heart failure, understand the priniciples of management and know when to refer

- Know the value of oxygen saturation measurement in the assessment of possible congenital heart disease

- Know the recommendations regarding endocarditis prophylaxis in children with heart diseases

References and Further Reading

1. Venugopalan P, Ranaweera M. Patient Management: Clinical Approach To Heart Murmurs In Children. Foundation Years Journal: 2014;8:20-3

2. Venugopalan P, Agarwal AK. Spectrum of congenital heart defects associated with Down Syndrome in high consanguineous Omani population. Indian pediatrics. 2003 May; 40(5):398-403

3. Centre for Clinical Practice at NICE, UK. Prophylaxis against infective endocarditis: antimicrobial prophylaxis against infective endocarditis in adults and children undergoing interventional procedures

4. Cowan, J. R., & Ware, S. M. (2015). Genetics and Genetic Testing in Congenital Heart Disease. Clinics in Perinatology, 42(2), 373–393

Chapter 15: Belly ache
Dr Thomas Whitby and Dr Gill Leonard

You are seeing patients in the paediatric gastroenterology out-patient clinic. Your first patient saw his GP 8 weeks ago and has the following referral letter;

"Please see Peter, a previously well 12 year old boy. His mother is worried that he has had a reduced appetite and been less energetic than usual. He admits to having abdominal pain for the past 6 weeks describing an intermittent, cramp-like pain in the lower abdomen. The pain is associated with nausea but is generally relieved by defecation. His stools are looser than usual but there is no blood or mucus. He denies any problems at home but did fall out with his best friend 2 months ago. On examination he appears well. His abdomen is soft with no palpable masses. His weight and height are growing along the 25th centile".

Q1. Which one of the following actions should the GP have done given this history?

A.   Abdominal X-ray
B.   Anti-Endomysial Antibody/Tissue Transglutaminase Antibody levels
C.   Abdominal ultrasound
D.   Reassurance
E.   Urgent referral to a gastroenterologist

Since being seen by his GP, Peter tells you that he has continued to have abdominal pain and diarrhoea. The pain is now worse on defecation and he has noticed blood in his stools. He has missed several days of school and he has lost 2 kg in weight.

On examination he is pale. His abdomen is tender on palpation in the lower quadrants. There are no palpable masses. An anal fissure is identified on external anal inspection.

Q2. Which one of the following investigations is most likely to provide a definitive diagnosis?

A.   Barium meal and follow through
B.   CT Abdomen
C.   Endoscopic biopsy
D.   ESR and CRP
E.   Faecal Calprotectin

You discuss with the consultant in clinic who commences Peter on glucocorticosteroids. However on review, it is noted that his growth is poor and he is experiencing unpleasant side effects. The steroids are stopped.

Q3. What would be your first line alternative treatment to induce remission?

A.   6-mercaptopurine
B.   Azathioprine
C.   Enteral nutrition
D.   Infliximab
E.   Methotrexate

Answers and Rationale

Q1.   D: Reassurance
Q2.   C: Endoscopic biopsy
Q3.   C: Enteral nutrition

When Peter first presents to his GP, no investigations are warranted since he has no "alarm symptoms" associated with his chronic abdominal pain. At this stage it was appropriate for Peter to be managed in primary care and he did not require a tertiary gastroenterology referral at his first presentation. Key "alarm symptoms" and signs are summarised in (Table 15.1). The presence of these features increases the probability of an organic disorder, such as inflammatory bowel disease, coeliac disease or other rare gastrointestinal pathologies. Patients with these alarm symptoms require further investigation and consideration of referral. In the 2 months Peter waited for his appointment he developed some of these alarm symptoms. The take home message of this scenario is the recognition of these alarm symptoms.

• Involuntary weight loss
• Linear growth deceleration
• Gastrointestinal blood loss
• Significant vomiting
• Chronic severe diarrhoea
• Persistent right sided abdominal pain
• Family history of inflammatory bowel disease
• Unexplained fever

Table 15.1: "Alarm symptoms" associated with chronic abdominal pain (1)

The aetiology of chronic abdominal pain in children is multifactorial and poorly understood. The prevalence of this condition is up to 20% in western countries. There are two age peaks, peaking at 4-6 years of age and then at 7-12 years of age. Most children with functional abdominal pain have relatively mild symptoms and are managed in primary care. The presence of life stresses or psyco-social difficulties are unhelpful in distinguishing between function and organic pathology (1).

The mainstay of treatment in children with chronic abdominal pain without "alarm symptoms" is reassurance. This includes family education and encouraging return to normal function rather than complete resolution of symptoms. However, the use of pharmacological treatment, such as analgesia, antispasmodics and probiotics may be used on an individual basis as part of a multifaceted management plan (1).

In the second question the clinical scenario has progressed. By the time Peter attends the gastroenterology clinic he now has features in keeping with an organic gastrointestinal disorder (Table 15.2). The weight loss, persistent worsening abdominal pain, chronic diarrhoea and blood in stool, peri-anal disease, along with systemic upset (pallor, arthralgia) should all be ringing alarm bells. These symptoms suggest an organic disease and further investigation is warranted. There are no nationally agreed absolute first line investigations. However as good practice most clinicians would undertake the following tests; FBC, ESR, CRP, Biochemistry, LFT Coeliac screen, Urine analysis, Stool MC+S and faecal colprotectin.

In this clinical case, inflammatory bowel disease (IBD) should be top of your list of differential diagnoses. Whilst some of his symptoms (e.g. abdominal pain, weight loss and chronic diarrhoea) can feature in other gastrointestinal disorders, such as coeliac disease or bowel malignancy, the presence of blood in stool and peri-anal disease suggests inflammatory bowel disease. His age is also in keeping with the median age of diagnosis being 12 years (3).

- Gastroesophageal reflux disease/eosophagitis
- Food intolerance (e.g., lactose maldigestion, fructose/sorbitol malabsorption)
- Coeliac disease
- Chronic inflammatory bowel disease (Crohn's disease, ulcerative colitis, indeterminate colitis)
- Peptic ulcer disease (in *Helicobacter* pylori infection)
- Pancreatitis
- Hepatobiliary diseases
- Anatomical malformations (e.g., Meckel diverticulum, malrotation, duplication)
- Neoplastic disease
- Dysmenorrhea
- Diseases of the urinary tract

Table 15.2: Common organic causes of chronic abdominal pain in childhood and adolescence (2)

The gold standard investigation to diagnose IBD is upper and lower GI endoscopies with serial mucosal biopsies.

A tissue diagnosis is essential. All the other investigations listed may be helpful but none are diagnostic. NICE now recommends faecal calprotectin testing in a person with suspected IBD. Faecal calprotectin is a substance released into the intestines in excess in the presence of inflammation (4). It is a useful test to help doctors distingish between inflammatory bowel diseases and non-inflammatory disorders. CRP and ESR are useful markers of infection and inflammation but neither are specific diagnostic investgiations. Further imaging such as a gadolinium – enhanced MRI, video capsule endoscopy and CT scan may be undertaken but again they do not provide a definite daignosis. A barium meal and follow through allows complete examination of the entire GI tract, in particular giving complete visualisation of the small bowel which is difficult to see on lower and upper endoscopy.

The final question focuses on the management of inflammatory bowel disease and more specifically Crohn's disease. It requires knowledge of the NICE guidelines (5). As with all chronic illnesses, management should be in a multidisciplinary setting overseen by tertiary services. The initial aim of management is to induce remission. NICE recommends that a child with their first presentation *or* a single inflammatory exacerbation of Crohn's in a 12 month period should be commenced on conventional glucocorticosteroids as first line monotherapy. Prednisolone, methylprednisolone or intravenous hydrocortisone are generally used. Budesonide may be used in distal ileal, ileocaecal or right-sided colonic disease in whom a conventional glucocorticosteroid is not appropriate. Budesonide is less effective than a conventional glucocorticosteroid but may have fewer side effects (4).

In this question the child is experiencing unwanted side effects from the steroids and remission has not yet been achieved. In this situation NICE recommends considering a 6 week exclusive enteral nutrition diet. There are two types of enteral nutrition: elemental (which is unpalatable and generally administered by NG-tube) and polymeric which is better tolerated orally. Systemic side effects are less than those for steroids but the remission duration is shorter. For a first presentation or a single inflammatory exacerbation in a 12 month period 5-aminosalicylate (5-ASA) can be considered in people who decline, cannot tolerate or in whom glucocorticosteroid treatment is contraindicated. 5-ASA is less effective than a conventional glucocorticosteroid but may have fewer side effects (4).

Where adequate control has not been achieved by first line therapy, add on therapy is required. Two or more inflammatory exacerbations in a 12 month period, or where glucocorticosteroid dose cannot be tapered suggests failure to induce adequate remission. The next step in management would be to consider adding azathioprine or mercaptopurine (4). Azathioprine is a pro-drug that is metabolised to 6-Mercaptopurine. It is a frequently prescribed immunomodulatory and may allow steroid sparing (3).

Syllabus Mapping

Gastroenterology and Hepatology (including surgical abdominal conditions)

- Know the causes of acute abdominal pain, and recognise when to refer, including urgency of referral

- Know the presentations, causes and management of chronic and recurrent abdominal pain including when to refer

- Know the causes of acute diarrhoeal illness, how to assess and manage and when to refer

- Know the common causes of upper and lower gastrointestinal bleeding, initial management and appropriate referral

References and Further Reading

1. Berger MY, Gieteling MJ, Benninga MA. Chronic abdominal pain in children. Bmj. 2007 May 12;334(7601):997-1002

2. Rasquin A, Di Lorenzo C, Forbes D, Guiraldes E, Hyams JS, Staiano A, Walker LS

3. Childhood functional gastrointestinal disorders: hild/adolescent.Gastroenterology. 2006 Apr; 130(5):1527-37

4. Gardiner M, Eisen S, Murpphy C. Training in Paediatrics the essential curriculum. Oxford University Press. 2009

5. Mayberry JF, Lobo A, Ford AC, Thomas A. NICE clinical guideline (CG152): the management of Crohn's disease in adults, children and young people. Alimentary pharmacology & therapeutics. 2013 Jan 1;37(2):195-203

6. Paediatric Formulary Committee. BNF for Children (BNFC) 2014-2015. Pharmaceutical Press; 2014 Jul 7

Chapter 16: A swollen face
Dr Louise Oni

Alfie is a 2 year old Caucasian boy who presents to the emergency department with a 3-day history of 'not being himself'. His mother reports that his face looks swollen and his abdomen is bigger than usual. The family have been unwell recently and he had a viral upper respiratory infection 1 week ago. His appetite is reduced but he continues to drink fluids well. He is not passing as much urine but he does not have any pain when passing urine. He has been taking paracetamol as required but no other medications.

On examination he is alert, warm well hydrated and well perfused. His heart rate is 110/minute and his blood pressure is 96/45 mmHg. He has facial oedema and bilateral pitting oedema to his ankles extending up to his knees. He has a distended, soft, non-tender abdomen

The urine dipstick shows protein++++, blood+, no nitrites and no leucocytes. He has investigations performed that confirm nephrotic syndrome and he is started on steroids. After a week of treatment he begins to respond.

Q1. What is the best test to confirm the diagnosis of nephrotic syndrome?

A. 24-hour urine protein collection
B. Renal ultrasound scan
C. Serum albumin and electrolytes
D. Urine microscopy and culture
E. Urine protein:creatinine ratio

Q2. If a renal biopsy were to be performed what is the most likely histological diagnosis?

A. C3 nephropathy
B. Focal segmental glomerulosclerosis
C. Lupus nephritis
D. Membranoproliferative glomerulonephritis
E. Minimal change disease

The following is a list of potential complications of childhood nephrotic syndrome:

A. Acute renal failure
B. Failure to respond to steroid treatment
C. Hyperlipidaemia
D. Hypertension
E. Hypothyroidism
F. Infection
G. Loss of skin integrity
H. Renal vein thrombosis
I. Sagittal sinus thrombosis
J. Tight scrotal oedema

For each of the following clinical situations select the most likely diagnosis:

Q3a. He develops a sudden onset of macroscopic haematuria with visible blood clots

Q3b. He has a severe headache that does not improve with simple analgesia

Q3c. Focal segmental glomerulonephritis is seen on the renal biopsy

Answers and Rationale

Q1. **C: Serum albumin and electrolytes**
Q2. **E: Minimal change disease**
Q3a. **H: Renal vein thrombosis**
Q3b **I: Sagittal sinus thrombosis**
Q3c **B: Failure to respond to steroid treatment**

Nephrotic syndrome is a triad of clinical oedema, heavy proteinuria ($>1g/m^2/day$) and hypoalbuminaemia ($<25g/L$) (1-3). A urine dipstick of 4+ protein is equivalent to approximately 5 grams per day of proteinuria, therefore heavy proteinuria is presumed in this scenario. A spot urine protein:creatinine ratio (or urine albumin:creatinine ratio) would be useful to help quantify the protein loss however 24-hour urine collections are rarely used in children as they are cumbersome. The best next test is the serum albumin as this would confirm hypoalbuminaemia as part of the triad for diagnosis.

Childhood nephrotic syndrome is classed as being 'typical' in children presenting between the ages of 1-10 years, with normal blood pressure, normal renal function and no macroscopic haematuria. In these 'typical' patients once baseline investigations have been performed, treatment with corticosteroids can empirically be started. A renal biopsy is not routinely indicated at presentation as previous studies have shown that patients who respond to corticosteroids within 4 weeks of treatment have a 90% chance of having minimal change disease histologically. Therefore the renal biopsy is reserved for those patients who do not respond to treatment or for those who present with 'atypical' features (aged <1 years or >10 years, hypertension, abnormal renal function and/or macroscopic haematuria). The most likely histological diagnosis in atypical cases is focal segmental glomerulonephritis (FSGS) and this generally carries a worse renal prognosis. Alternative causes of proteinuria can be seen in (Table 16.1).

Causes of Proteinuria Non-pathological:	Pathological
• Transient proteinuria • Fever induced • Exercise induced • Urinary tract infection • Postural proteinuria	• Nephrotic syndrome • Glomerulonephritis* • Chronic kidney disease • Tubular interstitial disease

*Table 16.1: Causes of non-pathological and pathological proteinuria in children (*see Table 16.3 for causes of glomerulonephritis)*

Complications of childhood nephrotic syndrome mainly arise due to hypovolaemia, thromboembolism or infection. Whilst children with nephrotic syndrome can present very oedematous and appear fluid overloaded, they are often intravascularly deplete which can make the clinical assessment of hydration status difficult. Signs of intravascular depletion include cool peripheries, increased core-peripheral temperature gap (>2 degrees) and tachycardia. The risk of thromboembolism is increased due to a reduced circulating volume and anti-thrombin III being lost in the urine producing a pro-thrombotic state. Thrombosis mostly occurs in the renal blood vessels (producing renal vein thrombosis; that presents as macroscopic haematuria often associated with abdominal pain) or the sagittal sinus venous system. The cerebral veins drain into the sagittal sinus system and thrombosis in this region presents as a worsening, unremitting headache occasionally with ophthalmic symptoms. Concerns about thromboembolism require urgent imaging and anticoagulation. Microscopic haematuria can be seen in typical cases and usually self resolves. Alternative causes of macroscopic haematuria include urinary tract infections and other causes of glomerulonephritis, as seen in (Table 16.2) (4). Macroscopic haematuria is an 'atypical' feature of childhood nephrotic syndrome and further investigations are required.

Causes of Haematuria	
• Urinary tract Infection	• Renal vein thrombosis
• Glomerulonephritis*	• Arteritis
• Urinary tract Stones	• Haematological disorder
• Trauma	• Drugs (e.g. cyclophosphamide)
• Renal tract tumour	• Exercise induced
• Polycystic kidney disease	• Fictitious

*Table 16.2: Causes of haematuria in children (*see Table 16.3 for causes of glomerulonephritis)*

There are several different types of glomerulonephritis that can be experienced in childhood; the most common of which are secondary to infection (5).(Table 16.3) details the causes of glomerulonephritis.

Causes of Glomerulonephritis Post Infectious:	Other
• Bacterial: streptococcal, staphyloccocu aureus, mycoplasma pneuomniae, salmonella	• Membranoproliferative glomerulonephritis
• Viral: herpes, EBV, varicella, CMV	• IgA nephropathy
• Fungi: candida, aspergillus	• Subacute bacterial endocarditis
• Parasitic: toxoplasma, malaria, schisosomiasis	• Shunt nephritis
	• Alports syndrome
	• Systemic Disease e.g. SLE

Table 16.3: Causes of glomerulonephritis in children

Syllabus Mapping

Nephro-urology

- Know the manifestations of acute and chronic renal diseases

- Know the causes of haematuria and proteinuria (including nephrotic syndrome and acute nephritis) and recognise features in the presentation which suggest serious or significant pathology

References

1. McCaffrey J, Lennon R, Webb NJ. The non-immunosuppressive management of childhood nephrotic syndrome. Pediatric Nephrology. 2015 Nov 10:1-20

2. Larkins N, Kim S, Craig J, Hodson E. Steroid-sensitive nephrotic syndrome: an evidence-based update of immunosuppressive treatment in children. Archives of disease in childhood. 2015 Aug 19:archdischild-2015

3. Suri D, Ahluwalia J, Saxena AK, Sodhi KS, Singh P, Mittal BR, Das R, Rawat A, Singh S. Thromboembolic complications in childhood nephrotic syndrome: a clinical profile. Clinical and experimental nephrology. 2014 Oct 1;18(5):803-13

4. Wood EG. Asymptomatic hematuria in childhood: a practical approach to evaluation. The Indian Journal of Pediatrics. 1999 Mar 1;66(2):207-14

5. Vinen, C. S., Oliveira, D. B. Acute glomerulonephritis. Postgrad Med J. 2003; 79, 206-213

Further Reading

Rees L, Brogan PA, Bockenhauer D, Webb NJA. Oxford specialist handbooks of Paediatrics: Paediatric Nephrology. Second edition. Oxford University Press 2012

Chapter 17: Out of control eczema
Dr Louise Cutts

(**17**)

Bala is a 5 year old boy who presents to the emergency department with a 2-day history of deterioration of his eczema. His parents explain he has been constantly scratching at his skin.

On examination he is miserable with cervical lymphadenopathy. He has a widespread erythematous and excoriated rash. There are also areas of vesicles, crusting and punched-out lesions mainly affecting his arms and legs and also some lesions in the periorbital area. His heart rate is 100/minute and temperature 36.4°C.

His parents have been applying regular emollients and hydrocortisone cream however this has failed to improve things. On further questioning, it is revealed that his sister has been suffering with a painful erosion of the upper lip.

Q1. Which is the most appropriate investigation to confirm a diagnosis of eczema herpeticum?

A.   Bacterial skin swab
B.   Full Blood Count (FBC)
C.   Serum HSV PCR
D.   Serum total IgE level
E.   Viral skin swab

Q2. What is the most important treatment for the above patient once a clinical diagnosis of eczema herpeticum has been made?

A.   Intravenous aciclovir
B.   Oral aciclovir
C.   Oral flucloxacillin
D.   Topical emollient cream
E.   Topical fusidic acid cream

Q3. Apart from the dermatology team, which of the following is the most important to be contatced for further assessment of this patient?

A.   Dermatology specialist nurse
B.   Health visitor
C.   Infection control nurse
D.   Ophthalmologist
E.   Paediatric on-call registrar

Answers and Rationale

Q1.   **E: Viral skin swab**
Q2.   **B: Oral aciclovir**
Q3.   **D: Ophthalmologist**

Eczema herpeticum is caused by an infection of the skin by the herpes simplex virus (HSV) which can be severe and potentially life-threatening. Infection with HSV 1 is more common than HSV 2. Children of all ages and ethnic groups can be affected and the highest incidence is in those aged 2-3 years. In most cases the patient is known to have a history of eczema (1). It usually presents as a deterioration of eczema accompanied by pain, lethargy and systemic upset. The rash of eczema herpeticum is vesicular often with crusting and punched out lesions that can coalesce. Any cutaneous site can be affected but most commonly there is involvement of the limbs. To confirm the diagnosis a viral swab should be taken and is the most important investigation when Bala first presents. Sensitivity is highest in the first 24-48 hours after an active vesicular lesion has appeared. Serum viral PCR is more sensitive and has good specificity but is not usually necessary due to cost implications (2). A bacterial swab should also be performed as co-infection with staphylococcus aureus can complicate eczema herpeticum.

Bala should be referred for an urgent dermatological opinion and treatment started immediately. The most important treatment is aciclovir. If the child is systemically unwell they should be admitted for intravenous aciclovir and fluid replacement. However, if the patient is systemically well aciclovir should be given orally. It is important to start aciclovir sooner rather than later and should be done so whilst awaiting virological confirmation. The recommended course duration for both intravenous and oral aciclovir is usually 5 days although sometimes longer courses are needed, and patients who are immunosuppressed require higher doses. Other supportive measures such as fluids and pain relief should also be instigated if necessary.

Clinicians are advised to be cautious with the use of topical steroids in eczema herpeticum as their use can potentially worsen the condition. Initial treatment should focus on anti-viral +/- antibacterial therapy. Periorbital involvement requires urgent referral to an ophthalmologist to look for corneal ulceration.

In children, atopic dermatitis or eczema is most commonly the earliest sign of atopy. This may be followed by allergic rhinitis, asthma and food allergy in the 'atopic march'. The discovery of "loss-of-function" mutations in genes encoding the protein filaggrin has led to a much greater understanding about the pathophysiology surrounding eczema (3). Filaggrin is an important epidermal protein expressed in the outer layers of the epidermis and plays a vital role in skin barrier function (4). Filaggrin gene mutations ultimately result in a deficiency of filaggrin and this is known to play a critical role in the development of atopic dermatitis (5). The clinical diagnosis of atopic dermatitis is based on a history of ill-defined itchy, dry, erythematous patches. These commonly affect flexural areas, although non-flexural areas are often affected especially in the young and there is commonly a family history of atopy.

Emollients

All children with atopic dermatitis should be offered the choice of un-perfumed emollients to use on a daily basis for moisturising, washing and bathing. They act by providing an effective barrier layer over the skin, decreasing moisture loss and protecting against irritants. There is a wide range available and choice should be suited to the child's needs and preferences with a combination being offered. Emollients should be prescribed in large quantities (250-500g weekly) and should be available at home, nursery and school.

Topical steroids

Topical steroids play an important part of treatment in eczema. They should be applied to areas of active eczema at the appropriate strength required to induce remission (6). A general rule is to use a topical steroid that settles eczema twice a day for 5-7 days and then reduce the frequency of application or potency. Areas of crusted or infected eczema may respond better to a steroid/antibiotic or a steroid/antiseptic combination. Local side effects, such as telangiectasia on cheeks and striae can be minimized if the appropriate steroid strength is used (7).

As a general rule:
- Use a mild potency steroid for mild atopic eczema i.e. hydrocortisone
- Use a moderate potency steroid for moderate atopic eczema i.e. Clobetasone butyrate 0.05%
- Use a potent steroid for severe atopic eczema i.e. betamethasone 0.1%

Other treatments

Topical calcineurin inhibitors (tacrolimus and pimecrolimus) are recommended as second or third-line agents in moderate to severe eczema and are licensed in patients aged 2 years and older. They do not cause skin thinning although those with a specialist interest in dermatology mostly prescribe them. Some patients may require regular application of dry or wet bandages to occlude topical treatments and help improve acute flare-ups. If available, this can be organised through a specialist department.

Psychosocial aspects

Moderate-severe eczema has a significant impact on quality of life of patients and their families. Itching, scratching and sleep deprivation can severely impair functioning and have a negative impact on psychosocial and psychological wellbeing (8). In addition regularly application of topical treatments is time-consuming. It is therefore important to educate patients and their carers about the importance of regular application of topical treatment to prevent flare-ups and avoidance of known triggers.

Syllabus Mapping

Dermatology

- Know the causes and management of skin infections and cellulitis

- Know the side effects and different potencies of topical steroids

- Be able to diagnose, investigate and manage common skin rashes e.g. eczema, acne, impetigo, staphylococcal scalded skin syndrome, dermatitis, cradle cap, and nappy rash

- Understand the emotional impact of severe dermatological problems

Ophthalmology

• Know the causes and management of eye infections and inflammatory disorders

References

1. Goodyear H M. Eczema Herpeticum Goodyear HM. Eczema herpeticum. Harper's Textbook of Pediatric Dermatology, 2 volume set. John Wiley & Sons, 2011

2. Moran PJ, Geoghegan P, Sexton DJ, O'Regan A. A skin rash to remember. BMJ 2012;345:e6625

3. Palmer CN, Irvine AD, Terron-Kwiatkowski A, Zhao Y, Liao H, Lee SP, Goudie DR, Sandilands A, Campbell LE, Smith FJ, O'Regan GM. Common loss-of-function variants of the epidermal barrier protein filaggrin are a major predisposing factor for atopic dermatitis. Nature genetics. 2006 Apr 1;38(4):441-6

4. Mclean WH Irwin and Irvine AD. Heritable filaggrin disorders: The paradigm of atopic dermatitis. Journal of Investigative Dermatology 2012;132(S3)E20-E21

5. Irvine AD, McLean WI, Leung DY. Filaggrin mutations associated with skin and allergic diseases. New England Journal of Medicine. 2011 Oct 6;365(14):1315-27

6. Brown S. Atopic eczema. Clinical Medicine 2016;16:66-69

7. Friedmann PS, Ardern-Jones MR and Holden CA. Atopic dermatitis. In: Burns T, Breathnach S, Cox N, Griffiths. Rook's Textbook of Dermatology 2010: 24.1-24.34

8. Atopic eczema in under 12's. NICE guidelines. https://www.nice.org.uk/guidance/cg57/chapter/1-Guidance (last accessed March 2016)

Further Reading

Irvine AD, Hoeger PH, Yan AC, editors. Harper's Textbook of Pediatric Dermatology, 2 Volume Set. John Wiley & Sons; 2011 Jul 28

Bruckner AL, Frieden IJ. Infantile Haemangiomas and Other Vascular Tumours. Harper's Textbook of Pediatric Dermatology, Volume 1, 2, Third Edition. 2006:113

Chapter 18: Vincent the vomiter
Dr Thomas Whitby and Dr Gill Leonard

Vincent is a 2 week old male presents to the GP with vomiting. He initially had a few vomits on the postnatal ward that were attributed to him being "mucousy". He was discharged at 24-hours bottle-feeding well. His parents have been concerned over the past week as he is bringing up some milk after feeds with winding. He is otherwise a contented baby. He takes 100 mls of formula milk every 3 hours and opens his bowels 2-3 times daily. He was born at term following an uneventful pregnancy. His birth weight was 3.95 kg and he now weighs 4.0 kg. On examination he is alert, well and hydrated and no abnormalities are detected.

Q1. What is the single most appropriate management plan for this baby?

A.   Reduce feed volumes
B.   Trail of alginate therapy
C.   Trial of feed-thickener
D.   Ultrasound scan of the abdomen
E.   Urine dipstick

He returns to the GP surgery at 5 weeks of age. His vomiting initially improved a little but he continued to bring up small to moderate amounts of milk after most feeds. He now weighs 5.3 kg and is taking 100 mls milk every 3 hours.

Q2. Which of the following is the most likely diagnosis?

A.   Cow's milk protein intolerance
B.   Gastro-oesophageal reflux
C.   Infantile hypertrophic pyloric stenosis
D.   Over-feeding
E.   Urinary tract infection

Vincent re-presents to the emergency department 1 week later with a further increase in his vomiting. His parents report that some of his vomits "have been hitting the wall" over the last 2 nights. The vomits are described as milky with no blood or bile staining. He is opening his bowels once a day. On examination he is mildly dehydrated. The clinician feels he has a normal abdominal examination. His weight today is 5.2 kg. As you are cannulating him, he has a forceful vomit, which travels approximately 1 metre, missing you but covering the medical student who is observing. A blood gas is sent to the laboratory and he is commenced on IV fluids.

Q3. Which of the following blood gas results would support the most likely clinical diagnosis?

A.   Hyperchloraemic hyperkalaemic metabolic alkalosis
B.   Hyperchloraemic hypokalaemic metabolic acidosis
C.   Hypochloraemic hyperkalaemic metabolic alkalosis
D.   Hypochloraemic hypokalaemic metabolic acidosis
E.   Hypochloraemic hypokalaemic metabolic alkalosis

Answers and Rationale

Q1. **A: Reduce feed volumes**
Q2. **B: Gastro-oesophageal reflux**
Q3. **E: Hypochloraemic hypokalaemic metabolic alkalosis**

Vomiting in babies is a common presenting complaint both in the community and secondary care. It is important that all clinicians can distinguish between posseting and vomiting. Posseting is a common normal occurrence. It happens after feeds when milk regurgitates into the oral cavity and out of the mouth. Vomiting on the other hand is a forceful contraction of the diaphragm and abdominal muscles and requires further exploration to elicit the underlying cause. It is essential to understand the significance of certain red flags. For example bilious vomiting should be presumed to be secondary to intestinal obstruction until proven otherwise. These babies can deteriorate quickly and therefore the clinician needs to be able to recognise an unwell, deteriorating infant both from the history and clinical examination. When Vincent first presents he is a well-baby (depicted by his weight gain, nature of the posseting and normal examination) who is being over fed. This infant is taking approximately 200ml/kg/day (recommended intake 150mls/kg/day). Therefore your first step in management would be to reduce the feed volumes as they are excessive for his weight. When he returns 3 weeks later he is now taking an appropriate amount of milk (150ml/Kg). On the basis that he is posseting small volumes frequently, gastro-oesophageal reflux (GOR) is now the most likely diagnosis. GOR is a normal physiological process in infancy and is characterised by the passage of gastric contents into the oesophagus. It affects approximately 40% of infants and typically occurs before 8 weeks of age. It does not require any investigation and can be managed by parental reassurance and advice (1). GOR that is associated with signs of distress or complications is referred to as gastro-oesophageal reflux disease (GORD). Associated risk factors for the development of GORD include prematurity, hiatus hernia, congenital diaphragmatic hernia, congenital oesophageal atresia and neurodisability. Complications of GORD include reflux oesophagitis, recurrent aspiration pneumonia, otitis media and dental erosion in children with neurodisabilities. In the majority of cases the management of GORD can be approached in a stepwise fashion. NICE recommends the following method in formulafed infants (1):

* Review the feeding history, **then**
* Reduce the feed volumes only if excessive for the infant's weight, **then**
* Offer a trial of smaller, more frequent feeds, **then**
* Offer a trial of thickened formula

In breastfed infants a breastfeeding assessment should initially be undertaken prior to any pharmacological treatment. If the above approaches are unsuccessful then you should consider a 1-2 week trail of alginate. If this helps, then the medication should be continued with regular breaks to see if the GOR has resolved. It is important to stop the feed thickener in bottle fed babies prior to commencing alginate therapy as the feeds would become too thick (1). If there is overt regurgitation with unexplained feeding difficulties, faltering growth or distressed behaviour then a 4-week trial of acid suppressing drugs, such as proton pump inhibitors (PPIs) or H_2 receptor antagonists (H₂RAs) should be considered (1).

In most cases no investigations are warranted. However if an infant has more sinister symptoms (Table 18.1) or the diagnosis is in doubt further investigations would be appropriate, usually under the guidance of a gastroenterologist.

Clinical features warranting investigation	
Oesophageal pH/Impendence study	**Upper GI endoscopy**
• Suspected recurrent aspiration pneumonia	• Haematemesis
• Unexplained nonepileptic seizurelike events	• Melaena
• Possible need for fundoplication	• Dysphagia
• A suspected diagnosis of Sandifer's syndrome	• No improvement in regurgitation after 1 year old
• Unexplained apnoeas	• Persistent, faltering growth associated with
• Unexplained upper airway	overt regurgitation
• inflammation	• Feeding aversion and a history of regurgitation
• Dental erosion associated with a neurodisability	• Unexplained iron deficiency anaemia
• Frequent otitis media	• A suspected diagnosis of Sandifer's syndrome

Table 18.1: Clinical indications for performing an oesophageal PH study/ Impedance study and an upper GI endoscopy in infants and young people (1)

A urinary tract infection should be considered in any infants with regurgitation if there is (1):
• Faltering growth
• Late onset (> 8 weeks)
• Frequent regurgitation and marked distress

Awareness of non-IgE mediated cows' milk protein allergy is an important differential in infants with symptoms of GORD. It is important to take a detailed history and assessment of any atopic symptoms, signs and/or a family history. Typically features of this condition occur in first four weeks of age. They include vomiting, failure to thrive, rash and proctocolitis. Most children outgrow food allergies by 2 to 4 years of age (3).

At 6 weeks of age Vinnie develops more impressive vomiting. The term "projectile vomiting" is often used by parents to describe large vomits, whereas the description of the vomit "hitting the wall" is useful and is indicative of infantile hypertrophic pyloric stenosis (IHPS). IHPS is the gradual hypertrophy of the pyloric muscular wall following the initiation of enteral feeding and can lead to obstruction of the pyloric lumen. The stenosis is not present at birth but evolves over the first few weeks. In IHPS the baby classically presents with recurrent projectile, non-bilious vomiting. They are usually hungry and constipation is common. Infants typically present between 2-6 weeks of age (but can present up to 12 weeks of age) with the male to female ratio being 4:1. The UK incidence is 1/1000 live birth (2). IHPS usually presents early, prior to clinically dehydration becoming apparent. There may be associated weight loss or poor weight gain. Abdominal examination may be normal, but visible peristaltic waves may be seen and a palpable pyloric mass may be felt during a "test feed" (2). In reality it is often difficult to detect a pyloric mass or peristaltic waves and most clinicians will instigate diagnostic investigations.

The gold standard investigation to diagnose IHPS is abdominal ultrasound. Muscle wall thickness >4mm and pyloric canal length >17mm is diagnostic (2). Blood gas classically demonstrates a hypochloraemic hypokalaemia metabolic alkalosis secondary to loss of the acidic gastric content in vomits (3). IHPS is not a surgical emergency. It is important to ensure the baby is adequately rehydrated and the electrolyte disturbance is corrected prior to theatre for definitive surgical treatment (Ramstedt pylormyotomy). The overall prognosis is excellent (3).

Syllabus Mapping

Gastroenterology and Hepatology (including surgical abdominal conditions)

- Know the causes of vomiting/regurgitation at different ages and be able to assess, manage and refer appropriately

- Know the common causes of food allergies and intolerances, their initial management and when to appropriately refer

- Be able to recognise and understand the management of common surgical conditions including hernias, and pyloric stenosis

Neonatology

- Know about the identification, initial management and appropriate referral pathways for neonatal surgical problems including NEC

References and Further Reading

1. NICE guideline No. 1. Gastro-oesophageal reflux disease in children and young people. 2015

2. BMJ Best Practice. Pyloric stenosis. http://bestpractice.bmj.com/best-practice/monograph/680.html (last accessed 10th March 2016)

3. Gardiner M, Eisen S, Murpphy C. Training in Paediatrics the essential curriculum. Oxford University Press. 2009

Chapter 19: To bolus, or not to bolus
Dr Rabin Mohanty

19

Nancy is a 10 year old girl who presents to the emergency department with her parents as she has been vomiting and is drowsy. Her parents tell you she has not been quite right for the past month and has been drinking a lot of water. They think she has lost some weight. There is no family history of diabetes.

On examination she has a heart rate of 150/minute, blood pressure of 100/60 mmHg and a respiratory rate of 25/minute with deep, labored breathing. Her capillary refill time is 3 seconds centrally. She responds to your voice but is drowsy. Her abdomen is generally tender to palpating. Her blood sugar is 32mmol/l and ketones are 7 mg/dl. Her venous blood gas is as follows;

pH	7.05
bicarbonate	9 mmol/l
pCO_2	3.2 KPa
base excess	-16

You make a diagnosis of type 1 diabetes presenting with diabetic ketoacidosis and send bloods for U&E, INR, Full Blood Count, HbA1c and ketones.

Q1. Which one of the following is the is best guide for you to decide about giving fluid bolus in this situation?

A. Base Excess
B. Blood pressure
C. Capillary refill time
D. Heart rate
E. Venous pH

Q2. Which one investigation might suggest that she is at higher risk of cerebral oedema?

A. High blood sugar
B. High INR
C. High white cell count
D. Low creatinine
E. Low pCO_2

Q3. What initial treatment is best if you suspect cerebral oedema?

A. Colloid infusion
B. Hypertonic saline
C. Hyperventilation with intubation
D. Increase potassium infusion
E. Stopping intravenous fluid

Answers and Rationale

Q1. **D: Heart rate**
Q2. **E: Low pCO$_2$**
Q3. **B: Hypertonic saline**

Nancy is presenting with classical symptoms and signs of diabetes culminating in an acute presentation with diabetic ketoacidosis (DKA). DKA is a medical emergency and the above scenario is a severe example. Severe DKA is defined when blood pH is <7.1 with DKA being mild to moderate if the pH is > 7.1 (1). There is controversy about giving fluid boluses to patients with DKA. Recent national guideline recommendations are not to give a fluid bolus unless the child is shocked which in Nancy's case is indicated by her tachycardia (2). Her capillary refill time of 3 seconds centrally may reflect the degree of acidosis causing vasoconstriction, rather than cardiogenic shock. Her blood pressure is within the normal range for her age. Her respiratory rate is elevated and laboured (Kussmaul's breathing) which is a physiological response aiming to reduce her pCO2 in an attempt to compensate for the metabolic acidosis.The management of DKA is initially the ABC approach, followed by rehydration and insulin therapy. 0.9% sodium chloride is the usual rehydration fluid with added potassium. In DKA there is always a massive depletion of total body potassium, irrespective of what the serum potassium level is (remember potassium is mainly an intracellular ion). The fluid correction of dehydration is done over a period of 48 hours during which time regular blood gases, glucose, electrolyte and neurological observations should be performed. Once rehydration fluids and potassium are running, blood glucose levels will start to fall. There is some evidence that cerebral oedema is more likely if insulin is started early and so national guidance is that insulin is commenced 1-2 hours after commencing the rehydration fluids (1). Cerebral oedema is a known complication during DKA management and has a mortality of around 25%. Signs and symptoms of this developing include altered consciousness, headache, agitation, high blood pressure, unequal pupils and abnormal posturing. The precise mechanism for the development of cerebral oedema is unknown. Risk factors for the development of cerebral oedema include younger age, receiving more than 40 ml/kg of fluid boluses and, low pCO2 levels (2). 3% hypertonic saline or 20% mannitol and early referral to an intensive care unit should be undertaken if there is suspicion of cerebral oedema. Hyperventilation with intubation is associated with an increased risk of cerebral oedema thought to be due to reperfusion following hypocapnic induced cerebral vasoconstriction. Further discussion on cerebral oedema in DKA is discussed in chapter 22.

Diabetes mellitus
Diabetes mellitus is a group of metabolic disease characterised by chronic hyperglycaemia resulting from defects in insulin secretion, insulin action or both. Around 70,000 children are diagnosed with diabetes every year. Finland, Sweden and Denmark have the highest rates of type 1 diabetes in the world. Type 1, type 2 and monogenic diabetes are the three major types described in children. 95% of children have type 1 diabetes (3). Type 1 diabetes is primarily due to an autoimmune T-cell mediated pancreatic islet beta cell destruction. Antibodies to islet cells (ICA), insulin (IAA) and other cellular components are present in 80-90% patients with type 1 diabetes. The inheritance of both HLA antigen DR3 and DR4 increases the risk of diabetes by 10 to 15 fold (4). Type 2 diabetes is rare in children with only 500 cases reported in the UK in 2013-14. It is suspected if symptoms occur in association with the

following; overweight/obesity, age > 10 years, strong family history, acanthosis nigricans, undetectable islet autoantibodies and elevated C-peptide (5). Metformin is commonly used to treat type 2 diabetes in children.

Around 1-4% children have monogenic diabetes. MODY (Maturity Onset Diabetes of Young) is inherited as autosomal dominant due to mutation of HNF gene. MODY 3 is most common where mutation occurs in the HNF1A gene. Young age of onset, strong family history of diabetes and low insulin requirements in non-obese children raises the suspicion of existence of MODY. UCPCR (Urine C-peptide Creatinine Ratio) is recommended for screening and the disease is confirmed by genetic test. Sulfonylurea is the drug of choice for HNF1-A MODY and HNF4-A MODY. Mutation of GCK gene causes very mild hyperglycaemia and does not need treatment. Renal cysts are associated with HNF1-B MODY (6).

Diagnosis of diabetes mellitus (3):
- Symptoms of diabetes plus random plasma glucose of ≥11.1 mol/l (200mg/dl) or
- Fasting (for at least 8 hours) plasma glucose ≥7.0 mmol/l or
- 2-hour post-load plasma glucose ≥11.1 mmol/l

Insulin regimes

The following are examples of the different insulin regimes used to treat diabetes;

(i)   2 injections of premixed insulin (both short and intermediate acting insulin)
(ii)   3 injections of premixed, short acting and long acting insulin
(iii) basal-bolus regime of long acting insulin in morning and night with short acting insulin with meals and
(iv)   Insulin pump therapy containing rapid acting insulin to stabilise variation in blood sugar with activity and food intake.

Carbohydrate counting is essential to calculate the dose of rapid acting insulin at meal times.

Screening in diabetes

Currently NICE recommends a target HbA1c as 48 mmol/ml (6.5%). There are several associated conditions and complications of diabetes which should be screened for on a regular basis (Table 1) Hypothyroidism is present in 3 - 8%, Coeliac disease in 1- 10% and Addison's disease in 1-2% in children with type 1 diabetes. NICE recommends screening for complications and associated conditions which is as follows (7):

Complications/ conditions	Time
Coeliac disease	At diagnosis
Thyroid disease	At diagnosis and annually
Retinopathy	Annually from the age of 12 years
Microalbuminuria	Annually from the age of 12 years
Blood pressure	Annually from the age of 12 years

Hypoglycaemia

Hypoglycaemia (blood sugar of ≤3.9 mmol/l) is the commonest acute complication in type 1 diabetes. Symptoms include headache, dizziness, nausea, blurred vision, trembling, seizure and coma. Mild to moderate hypoglycaemia can be treated with glucose tablets or juice or glucogel followed by slow acting carbohydrate if the child is not on insulin pump. Glucagon injection (0.5mg in children < 8 years or body weight < 25 kg and 1mg if > 8 years or > 25 kg) subcutaneously or intramuscularly is used to treat severe hypoglycaemia.

Causes of hypoglycaemia	
• Excessive bolus insulin dose	• Delayed effect of exercise
• Target levels set too low by patient or doctor	• Alcohol intake
• Illness	• Gastroparesis
• Excessive boluses being used to correct hyperglycaemia	• Basal rate too high in insulin pump
• Exercise without extra carbohydrate, or reduced bolus/basal insulin	• Infrequent blood glucose self-monitoring

Syllabus Mapping

Diabetes Mellitus

- Be able to recognise the features of a child or young person presenting with diabetes including diabetic ketoacidosis and know the principles of management

- Understand the management of diabetes in primary care including blood sugar monitoring and insulin regimens

- Know the causes, complications and treatment of hypoglycaemia in the diabetic child

Metabolism and Metabolic Medicine (including fluid management and acid base balance)

- Know about fluid, acid-base and electrolyte disturbances and their management

References and Further Reading

1. Glaser N, Barnett P, McCaslin I, Nelson D, Trainor J, Louie J, Kaufman F, Quayle K, Roback M, Malley R, Kuppermann N. Risk factors for cerebral edema in children with diabetic ketoacidosis. New England Journal of Medicine. 2001 Jan 25;344(4):264-9. National Paediatric Diabetes Report 2013-14

2. BSPED Recommended Guideline for the Management of Children and Young People under the age of 18 years with Diabetic Ketoacidosis 2015

3. National Paediatric Diabetes Report 2013-14. http://www.rcpch.ac.uk/system/files/protected/page/2014%20NPDA%20Report%201%202014%20FINAL.pdf. (Accessed on 10.04.2016)

4. Craig ME, Jefferies C, Dabelea D, Balde N, Seth A, Donaghue KC. Definition, epidemiology, and classification of diabetes in children and adolescents. Pediatric Diabetes 2014: 15 (Suppl. 20): 4-17

5. Zeitler P, Fu J, Tandon N, Nadeau K, Urakami T, Bartlett T, Maahs D. Type 2 diabetes in the child and adolescent. Pediatric Diabetes 2014: 15 (Suppl. 20): 26–46

6. Rubio-Cabezas O, Hattersley AT, Njølstad PR, Mlynarski W, Ellard S, White N, Chi DV, Craig ME. The diagnosis and management of monogenic diabetes in children and adolescents. Pediatric Diabetes 2014: 15 (Suppl. 20): 47–64

7. NICE Clinical Guidelines – NG18. Diabetes (type 1 and type 2) in children and young people: diagnosis and management, August 2015

Chapter 20: A busy Saturday in the emergency department
Dr Simon Li

You have rotated to the emergency department and it is your first weekend on call. In the morning 3 patients are brought in by ambulance.

This is a list of management options:

A.	Intramuscular adrenaline	F.	Intravenous mannitol
B.	Intravenous acyclovir	G.	Nebulised adrenaline
C.	Intravenous adrenaline	H.	Nebulised salbutamol
D.	Intravenous ceftriaxone	I.	Rectal diazepam
E.	Intravenous lorazepam	J.	Rectal paracetamol

Choose the most appropriate treatments for each of the following clinical scenarios:

Q1a. Amaya is a 5 year old girl with acute onset of shortness of breath commencing shortly soon after taking a first dose of penicillin V for tonsillitis. Her heart rate is 138/minute and respiratory rate 42/minute. On examination she has widespread blanching erythematous rash over his body and bilateral wheeze on auscultation.

Q1b. Barney is a 3 year old boy with cerebral palsy who is found collapsed at home. He is brought into the emergency department with basic life support in progress. Cardiac monitoring shows asystole.

Q1c. Chris is a 16 year old boy with a history of self-harm who presents unconscious with a heart rate of 154/minute, blood pressure of 168/103 mmHg and temperature of 39.4°C. Cardiac monitoring shows a broad-based tachyarrythmia. He is in possession of a bag of white powder.

Q2. Following Amaya's admission with suspected analyphylaxis to penicillin, what is the most appropriate discharge plan?

A.	Advise to avoid penicillin in future with no follow up required
B.	Advise to avoid penicillin and cephalosporins in future with no follow up required
C.	Prescribe an epinephrine auto-injection
D.	Provide a medical alert bracelet
E.	Refer to allergy specialist

Answers and Rationale

Q1a. **A: Intramuscular adrenaline**
Q1b. **C: Intravenous adrenaline**
Q1c. **E: Intravenous lorazepam**
Q2. **E: Refer to allergy specialist**

The assessment and management of the emergency situation is based upon the Advanced Paediatric Life Support (APLS) "ABCDE" structured approach which allows the rapid identification and management of key problems (1). Although somewhat artificial this is also true of scenarios in the theory examination, the only difference being that not all the parameters will be given to you. In any case it will be necessary to identify all the salient points from the case history to enable you to answer the question.

Amaya's symptoms of tachypnoea and tachycardia are temporally related to her taking a dose of penicillin. The blanching red rash and widespread wheeze support a diagnosis of a type 1 IgE-mediated hypersensitivity reaction to the penicillin which has led to urticaria and bronchospasm. Although it would not be futile to suggest nebulised salbutamol as the answer this can only be considered an adjunct as ultimately she requires a dose of intramuscular adrenaline (2). In this situation adrenaline has wide ranging actions including stimulation of; (i) alpha adrenoceptors which increases peripheral vascular resistance, reverses peripheral vasodilatation and reduction in angioedema; (ii) beta 1 adrenoceptors which have positive inotropic and chronotropic cardiac effects; and (iii) beta 2 adrenoceptors which causes bronchodilatation and reduces inflammatory mediator release. Although intravenous adrenaline can be used in difficult cases of anaphylaxis its use is restricted to intensive care settings (3).

Barney's case revises the management of the pulseless child. Algorithms are regularly updated by the Resuscitation Council UK (RCUK) and candidates are advised to revise their knowledge of all acute algorithms. In this situation, we have a child on the non-shockable side to the APLS algorithm (figure 20.1) with the management of asystole requiring effective chest compressions (with bag mask ventilation) until intravenous (or intraosseous) access is obtained to allow the administration of adrenaline. The right-hand side to figure (20.1) concerns the "shockable" rhythms, namely ventricular fibrillation and pulseless ventricular tachycardia. Children with these rhythms require DC cardioversion as well as effective cardiopulmonary resuscitation.

Chris' case is rather complex, though the above principles still apply. The fact that he has a history of self-harm would suggest that he has a history of risk taking behaviour and has ingested the white powder he is in possession of that has caused his current state. This ingestion has caused him to be unconscious, develop a tachyarrhythmia, hypertension and an elevated temperature. These features are in keeping with acute cocaine overdose whose management is largely symptomatic. Of primary concern are its deleterious effects on the cardiovascular system secondary to a hyperadrenergic state. After oxygenation this is managed with escalating doses of benzodiazepine. The hyperpyrexia in this situation is driven by the increased stimulation and activity of muscle causing heat production, together with vasoconstriction inhibiting heat loss.

Anaphylaxis from penicillin can be fatal and must be treated seriously. The possibility of a biphasic reaction means that children with a good response to initial treatment for suspected anaphylaxis should be observed for 6–12 hours. Blood samples for mast cell tryptase testing aids in determining if the event was indeed an anaphylactic reaction. Samples should be taken as soon as possible without delaying emergency treatment, one to two hours after the onset of symptoms and at least 24 hours later (4).

After emergency treatment for suspected anaphylaxis reaction a referral to a specialist allergy service should be made. A referral is NOT required for penicillin allergy. The specialist will ensure that the reaction was indeed anaphylaxis, provide education and also identify alternatives should they need antibiotics in future. Epinephrine injectors are not required as penicillin is easily avoided, as opposed to the inadvertent exposure of food allergens.

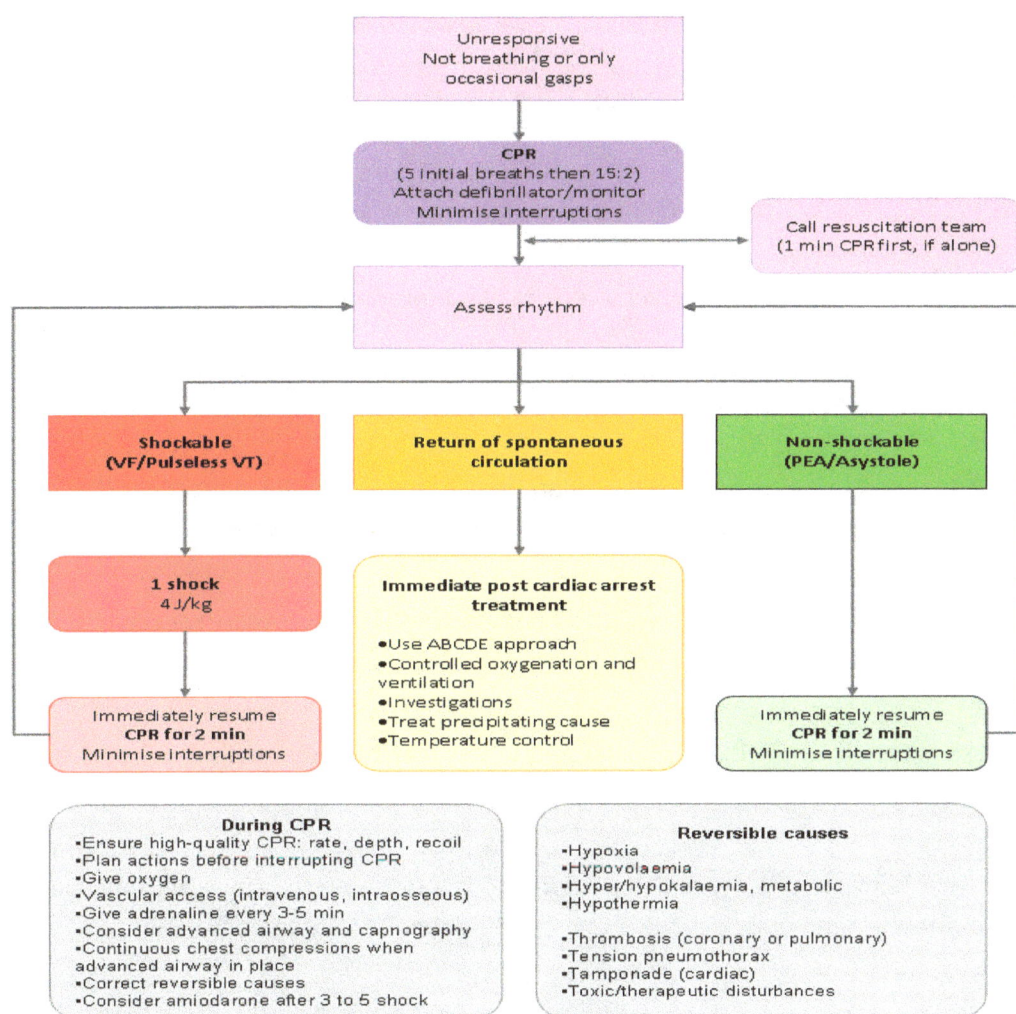

Figure 20.1: Advanced Paediatric Life Support Algorithm (Adapted from Resuscitation Council (UK) (5)**). CPR – cardiopulmonary resuscitation; VF – ventricular fibrillation; VT – ventricular tachycardia; PEA – pulseless electrical activity**

Syllabus Mapping

Emergency Medicine (including accidents and poisoning)

- Know the common causes of cardiac arrest, the prognostic factors that influence the outcome and how to provide basic life support and advise others.

- Be able to recognise and provide initial management for life-threatening airway, breathing or circulatory compromise

- Know the causes and features of anaphylaxis and its management

Infection, Immunology and Allergy

- Know the common allergies and advise on management

Pharmacology

- Know how to prescribe safely and be aware of adverse effects and interactions of drugs

References and Further Reading

1. Samuels M, Wieteska S, Advanced Life Support Group (Manchester England). Advanced paediatric life support : the practical approach. 5th ed. Chichester, West Sussex, UK: BMJ Books, 2011

2. Swan KE, Fitzsimons R, Boardman A, et al. The prevention and management of anaphylaxis. Paediatrics and Child Health 2012;22(7):264-71

3. Working Group of the Resuscitation Council (UK). Emergency treatment of anaphylactic reactions - Guidelines for healthcare providers, 2008

4. Anaphylaxis: assessment to confirm an anaphylactic episode and the decision to refer after emergency treatment for a suspected anaphylactic episode. NICE Clinical Guideline 134 December 2011

5. Maconochie I, B B, Skellet S. Paediatric advanced life support: Reuscitation Council (UK); 2015

Chapter 21: A busy Sunday in the emergency department

Dr Simon Li and Dr Chris Dewhurst

21

After Saturday's shift in Chapter 20 you contemplate a change in career. You spend Saturday night researching the training requirements of becoming a dolphin trainer. However you turn up for your shift on Sunday and the following children are brought in to the emergency department before 10 am.

This is a list of causes of raised intracranial pressure:

A.   Bacterial meningitis
B.   Brain tumour
C.   Cerebral abscess
D.   Cerebral oedema
E.   Herpes simplex encephalitis

F.   Hydrocephalus
G.   Idiopathic intracranial hypertension
H.   Ischaemic stroke
I.   Status epilepticus
J.   Subdural haemorrhage

Choose the most appropriate diagnosis for each of the following clinical scenarios:

Q1a. Ash is a 14 year old girl who presents unarousable and has a heart rate 64/minute with a blood pressure of 158/96 mmHg. She has the following results:

Blood glucose   34 mmol/l
Urinary ketones +++

Q1b. Ben is a 6 year old boy with cerebral palsy who is brought in by his foster carer and is obtunded. He was born at 24 weeks gestational age. His temperature is 37.3°C and is unarousable. He has a curvilinear scar to the left side of his skull.

Q1c. Cary is a 2 week old baby girl who presents as being lethargic and irritable. Her temperature is 36.9°C. On examination she has a bulging fontanelle and has circular bruises on both sides of her chest.

Initial blood results:

Haemoglobin	64 g/l	Platelets	254 x10^9/l
White cell count	8.3 x 10^9/l	CRP	5 mg/l

Q2. Which of the following clinical findings in a 2 year old child with suspected raised intracranial pressure is most concerning?

A.   Bradycardia
B.   Head circumference >99.6[th] centile
C.   Hyperreflexia
D.   Papilloedema
E.   Upward plantar response (positive Babinski sign)

Answers and Rationale

Q1a.   **D: Cerebral oedema**
Q1b.   **F: Hydrocephalus**
Q1c.   **J: Subdural haemorrhage**
Q2.   **A: Bradycardia**

As in chapter 20 the approach to the neurological emergencies is the structured "ABCDE" advanced paediatric life support approach (1).

In Ash's case there is evidence of impending tentorial herniation. Brain herniation is a life threatening complication of raised intracranial pressure and requires immediate neurosurgical intervention. You must therefore be vigilant for the early signs of impending herniation; the Cushing's triad of hypertension, irregular breathing and bradycardia. When herniation occurs decorticate posturing will frequently occur, with the elbows, wrists and fingers flexed, and legs extended and rotated inwards. In Ben's presentation whilst the other clinical findings are indicative of raised intracranial pressure they do not point to impending herniation. The extensor plantar response is a normal finding in infants, usually giving way to the flexor response at around 12 to 24 months of age.

What gives the game away as to the diagnosis in the Ash's presentation is that she is hyperglycaemic with elevated urinary ketones and thus is in diabetic ketoacidosis (DKA) secondary to her underlying type 1 diabetes. The treatment of children in DKA is intravenous fluid therapy and insulin (see chapter 19). Cerebral oedema is a much feared complication of children presenting in DKA. It was originally thought that over judicious fluid resuscitation leads to cerebral oedema as a result of osmotic changes and fluid shifts that occur during the treatment of DKA. However, through serial cranial CT studies have shown that subclinical cerebral oedema already exists in many DKA cases with no demonstrable link between treatments and developing DKA associated cerebral oedema (2). There have even been instances reported in the literature of DKA associated cerebral oedema before any possible treatment effect, as is the case in this instance in question 1 (3). Whilst the link between fluid resuscitation and the development of cerebral oedema remains controversial, the most recent guidance reflects a cautious approach to fluid administration (4).

Given the improvements in the treatment of extremely premature infants and children with serious illnesses, the number of children presenting for medical attention with co-existing morbidities is increasing and Ben's case highlights this point. The extreme prematurity and curvilinear scar point to a ventriculo-peritoneal (VP) shunt being in-situ. It is likely that the hydrocephalus is secondary to a significant intraventricular bleed in the neonatal period. A VP shunt is a device that removes excess cerebrospinal fluid (CSF) from the brain to the peritoneal cavity in children with hydrocephalus. Children with a VP shunt are just as likely to contract the usual array of childhood illnesses however an awareness of the VP shunt is necessary as complications with the shunt may be the underlying cause of their symptoms. Children with fever should be examined like any other child and a source for their fever found by excluding the usual suspects (chest, urine, ENT etc.). If however these are negative then an infected VP shunt must be high on the differential diagnosis. Antibiotics to cover for a CNS infection along with discussion with the neurosurgical team will be required (5).

The other concern to be aware of with VP shunts is its potential to become blocked. In Ben's case the shunt has become blocked leading to the build-up of CSF within the brain with subsequent hydrocephalus and raised intracranial pressure. Part of the VP shunt called the Ommaya reservoir will be palpable on examination. This is an access device which provides the facility for aspiration of CSF in situations of acutely raised ICP by a suitably trained clinician. The diagnosis of a blocked VP shunt is suspected when the Ommaya reservoir is unable to be depressed. When such a diagnosis is suspected discussion with a neurosurgeon and urgent CT scan of the head is required (5).

Paediatricians are often suspicious characters and we, when faced with any child, must be mindful that a child's welfare is paramount and be aware of safeguarding concerns. Infants presenting within the first weeks of life who are irritable on handling may have meningitis which can only be diagnosed on lumbar puncture and cerebrospinal fluid analysis. However this possibility would seem unlikely when Cary presents given that her temperature is normal, with an unremarkable white cell count and CRP. More concerning in a child of this age are the bruises which raises concerns about physical abuse, presumably from fingertip marks. Add in the fact she has haemoglobin of 64 which, even for a neonate undergoing normal physiological anaemia is very low, the concern would be that she has suffered an intracranial bleed. A CT scan of her brain should be requested to confirm the diagnosis and full child protection procedures initiated once confirmed which includes a skeletal survey, ophthalmological examination and blood tests.

Syllabus Mapping

Emergency Medicine (including accidents and poisoning)

- Know how to recognise acute seizures and initiate emergency treatment

- Know how to recognise and initiate treatment for children presenting with neurological emergencies

Neonatology

- Know the problems associated with prematurity and the long-term sequelae including the impact on the family and community

Neurology

- Know the likely causes and management of meningitis/encephalitis and altered consciousness

Safeguarding

- Know the presentations of physical, emotional and sexual abuse, neglect and fabricated and induced illness

References and Further Reading

1. Samuels M, Wieteska S, Advanced Life Support Group (Manchester England). *Advanced paediatric life support : the practical approach*. 5th ed. Chichester, West Sussex, UK: BMJ Books, 2011

2. Brown TB. Cerebral oedema in childhood diabetic ketoacidosis: is treatment a factor? Emerg Med J 2004;**21**(2):141-4

3. Glasgow AM. Devastating cerebral edema in diabetic ketoacidosis before therapy. Diabetes care 1991;**14**(1):77-8

4. National Institute for H, Care E. *Diabetes (Type 1 and Type 2) in Children and Young People: Diagnosis and Management*. London: NICE, 2015

5. Pettorini B, Williams D. The unwell child with a ventriculo-peritoneal shunt. Paediatrics and Child Health 2015;**25**(11):533-34

Chapter 22: A bottom shuffling boy
Dr Michelle Arora and Dr Kamath Tallur

22

John is a 20 month old boy who is referred to clinic by the health visitor due to concerns about his development. He was rolling at 4 months and sitting without support at 8 months. He now mobilises by "bottom shuffling". He was born at term by vaginal delivery. His mother has poorly controlled epilepsy and took antiepileptic medication during pregnancy. He has 2 older half-siblings who have no health problems with 1 sibling walking by 14 months and the other by 16 months. His father also bottom shuffled.

His head circumference, weight and length are on the 50th centile. He has symmetrically reduced tone, power and reflexes in both lower limbs. Upper limb examination is normal. There are no dysmorphic features or neurocutaneous features. Examination with Wood's light reveals no areas of hypopigmentation.

He has difficulty standing without support and is unable to walk but you observe him bottom shuffling. He can build a tower of 4 cubes and can scribble with a pencil using his right hand. He can say about 15 words with meaning and responds to his own name. There are no concerns about his hearing or vision. His mother says he feeds himself finger food and with a spoon and enjoys throwing balls.

His GP had performed a full blood count, renal function, liver function, creatine kinase and ferritin prior to referral. These are all within the normal range.

Q1. Which area of his development is delayed?

A.   Fine motor
B.   Global developmental delay
C.   Gross Motor
D.   Social, emotional and behavioural
E.   Speech and language

Q2. In reviewing this case, when should John have been referred for further assessment and/or investigation?

A.   When he only spoke 15 words by 20 months
B.   When he first demonstrated bottom shuffling
C.   When he was not rolling by 3 months
D.   When he was not sitting by 7 months
E.   When he was not walking by 18 months

Q3. What is the best diagnostic investigation for this child?

A.   Chromosomal analysis
B.   Hearing assessment
C.   MRI head and spine
D.   Serum amino acids and urine organic and amino acids
E.   Thyroid function tests

Answers and Rationale

Q1. **C: Gross motor**
Q2. **E: When he was not walking by 18 months**
Q3. **C: MRI head and spine**

The main areas of development are:

- Gross motor
- Vision and fine motor
- Hearing, speech and language
- Social, emotional and behavioural

Children develop at different rates, and it is important to distinguish those who are within the "normal" range from those who are delayed. Developmental delay is defined as being at least 2 standard deviations below the mean during developmental testing on an age appropriate standardised norm-referenced test and is estimated to be prevalent in 1-3% of children less than 5 years old (1).

Delay might be identified through routine screening, or by relatives, school, nursery or health professionals. Early identification is important as it allows early intervention and improves the outcome of children with developmental impairments (2). Table 22.1 indicates a list of red flags which should prompt consideration of further investigation (3).

Assessment can be performed in children under 5 years old using a range of tools, such as the Schedule of Growing Skills, the Griffiths Mental Development Scales or the Bayley Scales of Infant Development. Accurately assessing which stage the child scores in each of these parameters can help aid early diagnosis and identify what further input is needed. They can also reassure parents or carers if the child's development falls within normal limits. School age children can be assessed using the Wechsler Intelligence Scale for Children or the British Abilities Scales 2nd Edition (1997). It is useful to repeat developmental assessments to monitor developmental progress compared to chronological age.

In this scenario, John is unable to walk at 18 months. He therefore has delayed gross motor development. Approximately 9% of children will bottom shuffle instead of crawl. Bottom shufflers often have a family history of bottom shuffling and/or low muscle tone, as in John's case. While bottom shufflers tend to walk unsupported slightly later (at around 17-24 months) than non-bottom shufflers, assessment is still recommended for children who are not walking at 18 months to consider pathological cause (4).

Investigations aim to identify pathological causes for developmental delay, such as structural brain abnormalities, genetic abnormalities or metabolic problems such as thyroid disorders and inborn errors of metabolism. However, investigations should be tailored according to the history and examination findings (5,6). In a male child with delayed walking it is important to consider Duchenne's muscular dystrophy (DMD). Prompt diagnosis and treatment is imperative, as complications include progressive difficulty walking, dilated cardiomyopathy, arrhythmias and respiratory failure.

When you examine John you identify reduced tone, power and reflexes of his lower limbs bilaterally, indicating a likely lower motor neurone lesion. Hypotonia and reduced power may be a feature of DMD at this age but the reduced reflexes are not in keeping with this diagnosis. The normal creatine kinase excludes DMD. Developmental dysplasia of the hips can sometimes be missed on newborn postnatal check and not detected until the child presents with delayed walking. However, you would not expect to find hypotonia and hyporeflexia in such cases.

John had antenatal exposure to anti-epileptic drugs and was also an unplanned pregnancy, meaning it was unlikely that his mother was taking folic acid at conception. The likelihood of a neural tube defect is therefore increased and this would fit with the clinical findings. MRI of the spine may detect spina bifida occulta with brain scanning required to detect any potential additional complications including hydrocephalus and Arnold-Chiari malformation.

Positive indicators (the presence of the following):
<ul><li>Loss of developmental skills at any age</li><li>Parental of professional concerns about vision, fixing or following; or confirmed visual impairment at any age (simultaneous referral to paediatric ophthalmology)</li><li>Hearing loss at any age (simultaneous referral for expert audiological or ear, nose and throat assessment)</li><li>Persistently low muscle tone or floppiness</li><li>No speech by 18 months, especially if the child does not try to communicate by other means such as gestures (simultaneous referral for urgent hearing test)</li><li>Asymmetry of movement or other features suggestive of cerebral palsy, such as increased muscle tone</li><li>Persistent toe walking</li><li>Complex disabilities</li><li>Head circumference above the 99.6th centile or below the 0.4th centile, or circumference crossing two centiles (up or down) on the appropriate chart or is disproportionate to parental head circumference</li><li>An assessing clinician who is uncertain about any aspect of development but thinks the development may be disordered</li></ul>
Negative indicators (activities that the child cannot do):
<ul><li>Sit unsupported by 12 months</li><li>Walking by 18 months (boys) or 2 years (girls) (check creatine kinase urgently)</li><li>Walk other than on tiptoes</li><li>Run by 2.5 years</li><li>Hold objects placed in hand by 5 years (corrected for gestational age)</li><li>Reach for objects by 6 months (corrected for gestational age)</li><li>Point at objects to share interest with others by 2 years</li></ul>

Table 22.1: Red flags in development indicating further assessment/investigation (3)

Disability can have a considerable impact on families and carers and a multidisciplinary approach is vital in managing patients with spina bifida. Input from physiotherapy, urology and occupational therapy can improve the child's quality of life. The child may also need adaptions to accommodate him at home and nursery or school.

Syllabus Mapping

Musculoskeletal

- Be aware of the presentation of muscular disease including the dystrophies

Neonatology

- Know and understand the effects of antenatal and perinatal events

Neurodevelopment and Neurodisability

- Understand normal development including common variants

- Know the causes of disability, disordered development and learning difficulties

- Understand the definition and effects of neurodisability on children and families

References

1. Dorling J, Salt A. Evidence based case report: Assessing developmental delay. BMJ 2001 21;23(7305): 148–149

2. Gomby DS, Larner MB, Stevenson CS, Lewit EM, Behrman RE. Long term outcomes of early childhood programs: analysis and recommendations. Future Child 1995;5:6-2

3. Horridge KA. Assessment and investigation of the child with disordered development. Archives of disease in childhood-Education & practice edition. 2011 Feb 1;96(1):9-20

4. Sharma A, Cockerill H. Mary Sheridan's from Birth to Five Years: Children's Developmental Progress. 4th ed. Routledge. 2014

5. Shevall M, Ashwal S, Donley D, Flint J, Gingold M, Hirtz D, Majnemer A, Noetzel M, Sheth RD. Practice parameters: Evaluation of a child with global developmental delay: Report of the Quality Standards Subcommittee of the American Academy of Neurology and The Practice Committee of the Child Neurology Society. Neurology 2003; 60: 367-380

6. McDonald L, Rennie A, Tolmie J, Galloway P, McWilliam R. Investigation of global developmental delay. Archives of disease in childhood. 2006 Aug 1;91(8):701-5

Further Reading

Development Matters in the Early Years Foundation Stage (EYFS). The British Association for Early Childhood Education. London. 2012. (found at http://www.foundationyears.org.uk/files/2012/03/Development-Matters-FINAL-PRINT-AMENDED.pdf accessed March 2016)

Chapter 23: Stopping the seizure
Dr Rachel Varughese and Dr Anna Mathew

(23)

Sarah is an 8 year old girl who has epilepsy and is having outpatient follow up. She has had 2 admissions for prolonged seizures in the past 4 months. Her background regular medication has been adjusted but her mother is concerned about her having seizures at home. Your consultant has asked you to prescribe a supply of 4 doses of a rescue medication that may be used in the event of a seizure at home.

Sarah is otherwise well, with a recent weight of 25 kg. She is well kempt and is happy and outgoing during the consultation.

Q1. Given the scenario what would be the most appropriate rescue medication?

A.   Buccal midazolam, dose calculated by age
B.   Buccal midazolam, dose calculated by weight
C.   Extra doses of Sarah's regular epilepsy medication
D.   Rectal Diazepam, dose calculated by age
E.   Rectal Diazepam, dose calculated by weight

Q2. Which of the following would be necessary to include in the prescription?

A.   Sarah's age and weight
B.   The dose of the medication written in words and figures
C.   The name of the caregiver who will be administering the medication
D.   The pharmacy from which to collect the medication
E.   The total quantity of the medication prescribed written in words

Q3. What is the most important information should you give Sarah's parents about midazolam?

A.   Continue to administer one dose every 10 minutes until seizure activity stops
B.   Give midazolam as soon as there is evidence of a seizure starting
C.   Midazolam should only be given in generalised tonic clonic seizures
D.   Storage should be an easy to reach place, such as the family fridge
E.   Wait 5 minutes from the onset of the seizure before administering midazolam

Answers and Rationale

Q1: A: Buccal midazolam, dose calculated by age
Q2: B: The dose of the medication written in words and figures
Q3: E: Wait 5 minutes from the onset of the seizure before administering midazolam

In children with epilepsy, a history of prolonged seizures should be a prompt to consider prescribing rescue medication. The timely administration of medication to terminate a seizure can prevent progression to status epilepticus and potential long-term neurological damage.

Regular epilepsy medication is dosed and licensed for baseline control, and would therefore be inappropriate to prescribe as a rescue medication. A short acting drug, such as a benzodiazepine, is most appropriate in this case. Both midazolam and diazepam are members of the benzodiazepine family of drugs, and both are licensed for use in epilepsy in children. They enhance the effect of GABA (y-aminobutyric acid) on GABA receptors, leading to neural inhibition.

Midazolam is administered as a liquid rescue medication into the buccal cavity. It is accepted that buccal midazolam should be viewed as an effective and safe first line therapy in children requiring rescue medication in epilepsy. The buccal route is preferred to oral, as it allows rapid absorption across the buccal membrane, avoiding first-pass hepatic metabolism (1).

In this scenario, rectal diazepam is also a possibility, and this was historically the gold standard of treatment. However, it can be difficult to administer depending on the position of the child during the seizure or if the child is constipated, and is now considered less socially acceptable due to the administration route. In addition, if the bowels open after administration, it can be difficult to determine what dose has been delivered. It has also been shown to have a longer response time when compared to buccal midazolam and a less predictable absorption profile (1).

The dose of midazolam is calculated by age and not by weight. The BNFC (British National Formulary for Children) contains dosing and preparation information. This should be considered a vital tool in informing and confirming safe prescribing. For a child aged 5-9 years the dose is 7.5mg, for example one Buccolam 7.5mg/1.5ml oromucosal solution pre-filled oral syringe (2).

With administration of midazolam for seizure cessation caregivers should be advised to:

1. Wait five minutes from the onset of the seizure before administering midazolam
2. Call an ambulance if the seizure has not slowed or stopped after a further five minutes
3. Call an ambulance if they are unable to give the medication
4. Call an ambulance if there are b5reathing difficulties following administering the drug, for example blue lips, not breathing
5. NOT administer more than one dose at home

The buccal cavity can be described as the space between the inside of the cheek and the teeth, which is important for quick absorption. Since the medication comes in pre-filled syringes, parents should know that the full syringe contains the exact dose required.

Midazolam is a benzodiazepine, and is classed as a controlled drug. The Misuse of Drugs Act 1971 (3) sets out regulations for drugs considered to be potentially harmful or with potential for misuse. Since many of these drugs have legitimate uses within medicine, these regulations set out controlled rules on prescribing, administration, dispensing, documentation and custody of controlled drugs. Midazolam is licensed for children in status epilepticus, but not for adults. When prescribing any medication it is important to check that it is licensed for the use intended in the current prescription. The licence for a medication defines important characteristics about how it should be used, including indications, contraindications and dosing. The presence of a licence indicates that medication has undergone assessment for efficacy, safety and quality in the patient group that it is licensed for. The licence may specify a number of qualifying factors including age range, gender or diagnosis. Using a medication off license, means that the prescriber has deemed an unlicensed medication to be in the best interests of the patient, supported by available evidence. Using a medication 'off label' means using a licensed medication outside of the terms of its license (4).

Since comparatively fewer clinical pharmaceutical trials involve children as compared to adults, the most common scenario for 'off label' prescribing in paediatrics involves using a medication outside of the age range that it is licensed for. Prescribing unlicensed medicines or licensed medicines for unlicensed uses changes the professional liability of the prescribing doctor, and extra justifications must be made.

For a controlled drug, the prescription must contain:

1. The full name, date of birth and address of the patient
2. The name and formulation of the drug, even if only one form exists
3. The strength of the preparation
4. The dose in **both words and figures**
5. The total quantity in **both words and figures**
6. Prescriber signature, date and prescriber address

Safe prescribing is a hallmark of a good doctor and the GMC's Good Medical Practice highlights some key areas pertinent to prescribing (5). Errors within healthcare are often multifaceted, with human error acting as a common contributor. In the UK, prescribing errors occur in 1.5% of prescriptions, excluding near-misses, and there is some evidence that errors and harm is greater in children (6). Paediatricians face an especially difficult situation due to the age range of their patients; many medications are not licensed in certain paediatric age groups and doses vary widely, determined by age, body surface area, clinical condition or weight (7).

Prescribers must work within the limits of their knowledge and if tasked with a job that is beyond their experience, senior support or pharmacist advice must be sought. Many clinical incidents are due to poor prescribing and prescribing errors can be fatal. Prescribers of controlled drugs have a responsibility to ensure their choice of medication is necessary and safe for the patient. Clear documentation must be made in the notes as to the justification of the prescription.

When prescribing a controlled drug for parents to administer at home, it is important to provide clear instructions on how to administer the medication. Verbal instructions should not suffice, ideally, clear written information leaflets should be provided. In addition, adequate training must be given to ensure caregivers have confidence on when and how to administer medications. The PERFECT study highlighted deficiencies in the guidance given to caregivers, resulting in under-confidence and misunderstanding of administration (8).

Advice regarding storage of the medication is vital. Parents should be told to keep the medicine in its original packaging in a cupboard, away from heat and direct sunlight. Children should not be able to see or reach the medicine. It is necessary to have understanding of the major side effects, and to communicate these to parents in a sensitive and clear way. Profound sedation, respiratory depression, disinhibition and restlessness may all occur with benzodiazepines. There is a real but rare risk of respiratory arrest, which must be discussed with parents.

Syllabus Mapping

Pharmacology

- Know how to find out information necessary for safe prescribing through use of paediatric formularies and pharmacy liaison

- Know how to prescribe safely and be aware of adverse effects and interactions of drugs

- Know about the need to explain to parents the unlicensed and off-label prescription of drugs

References and Further Reading

1. Dean B, Schachter M, Vincent C, Barber N. Prescribing errors in hospital inpatients: their incidence and clinical significance. Quality and Safety in Health Care. 2002 Dec 1;11(4):340-4

2. Paediatric Formulary Committee. BNF for Children (BNFC) 2014-2015. Pharmaceutical Press; 2014 Jul 7

3. Misuse of Drugs Act, 1971 c.38. http://www.legislation.gov.uk/ukpga/1971/38 (accessed 21st March 2016)

4. Medicines and Healthcare products Regulatory Agency. Drug Safety Update; Off-label or unlicensed use of medicines: prescribers' responsibilities. 2009 April 1. https://www.gov.uk/drug-safety-update/off-label-or-unlicensed-use-of-medicines-prescribers-responsibilities (accessed 26th June 2016)

5. General Medical Council. Good practice in prescribing and managing medicines and devices. 2013. http://www.gmc-uk.org/guidance/ethical_guidance/14316.asp. (accessed 21st March 2016)

6. Kaushal R, Bates DW, Landrigan C, McKenna KJ, Clapp MD, Federico F, Goldmann DA. Medication errors and adverse drug events in pediatric inpatients. Jama. 2001 Apr 25;285(16):2114-20

7. Wong IC, Ghaleb MA, Franklin BD, Barber N. Incidence and nature of dosing errors in paediatric medications. Drug Safety. 2004 Aug 1;27(9):661-70

8. Arzimanoglou A, Lagae L, Cross JH, Beghi E, Mifsud J, Bennett C, Schmidt D, Wait S, Harvey G. The administration of rescue medication to children with prolonged acute convulsive seizures in a non-hospital setting: an exploratory survey of healthcare professionals' perspectives. European journal of pediatrics. 2014 Jun 1;173(6):773-9

Chapter 24: Hot headaches
Dr Jim Gould

Your rotation in the emergency department continues to be busy. On your next shift in the department the nurse practitioner hands over 3 children.

Here is a list of bacteria producing infection in children:

A.	Bacteroides	F.	Salmonella typhimuium
B.	Klebsiella pneumoniae (aerogenes)	G.	Staphylococcus aureus
C.	Mycobacterium tubercaulosis	H.	Streptococcus anginosis (Group H Strep)
D.	Mycoplasma pneumoniae	I.	Streptococcus pyogenes (Group A Strep.)
E.	Pseudomonas aeruginosa	J.	Streptococcus pneumoniae (pneumococcus)

Choose the most likely bacterium causing sepsis for each of the following children:

Q1a. Millie is a 12 year old girl with a 48 hour history of low grade fever, dry unproductive cough and a headache. She has recently moved to the UK from Portugal. She has a temperature of 38,8°C, respiratory rate 35/minute, heart rate 135/minute, blood pressure 85/65 mmHg and a capillary refill time <2 seconds.On examination she has absent breath sounds at the left base with no added sounds. There is dullness to percussion at the left base.

Q1b. Annie is a 14 year old girl, with a 4 day history of discomfort and puffyness of the tissues around her right eye. In the last 48 hours she has had a low grade fever and headache and more recently she has complained of bright lights hurting her eyes. She has recently been on holiday to Egypt. Her temperature is 38.2°C, heart rate 140/minute, blood pressure 140/85 mmHg, respiratory rate 25/minute, and capillary refill time of <2 secs. On examination she has erythema and swelling around the right eye which is tender. She has marked neck stiffness and although she was able to obey verbal commands she will not speak. Examination of her fundi shows bilateral papilloedema.

Q1c. Andis is a 5 year old boy who has been brought into the department by ambulance after having a seizure. He has a 3-week history of listlessness, poor appetite and low grade intermittent fever and before the seizure complained of a headache. He has recently moved to the UK from Latvia. His temperature is 38.2°C, heart rate 100/minute, respiratory rate 26/minute, blood pressure 85/50 mmHg and capillary refill time of < 2 seconds. On examination he has lymphadenopathy in the left jugulodigastric region and neck stiffness. His pupils are unequal, his left pupil being larger than the right and reacting sluggishly to light, with he had a left proptosis, both fundi appeared to be normal.

Q2. The main purpose of the UK notification system is to:

A.	Assist in planning ways to prevent future infection outbreaks
B.	Back up confirmatory data from the laboratories
C.	Detect and intervene in possible epidemic disease
D.	Improve the accuracy of diagnosis
E.	Monitor diseases imported from overseas

Answers and Rationale

Q1a.   **J: Streptococcus pneumoniae (pneumococcus)**
Q1b.   **H: Streptococcus anginosis (Group H Strep)**
Q1c.   **C: Mycobacterium tuberculosis**
Q2.   **C: Detect and intervene in possible epidemic disease**

Parapneumonic empyema

The history and findings in Millie's case strongly suggests an empyema in the pleural space rather than a simple effusion, and the aetiology is likely to relate to an underlying pneumonia. The presence of pus could be confirmed by a pleural tap. Management of pleural empyemas of any significant size will always require drainage as well as antibiotics. Because of loculation within the empyema space and the viscosity of the fluid, a large chest drain with instillation of a fibrinolytic agent was standard treatment but in most centres videoscopic-assisted thoracoscopy surgery (VATS) is now the preferred option (1). Organisms are often seen on gram film of the fluid, but quite often not grown on culture, as the child will often have been on antibiotic for some days prior to the procedure. Nevertheless, the commonest infecting agent in the UK and most countries by far is *Streptococcus pneumoniae* which, in the UK at least, usually remains sensitive to high dose systemic penicillin. Other organisms including *S. pyogenes* and *Staph. aureus* are sometimes seen, and potentially any of the organisms on the list can produce a parapneumonic empyema. With the introduction of the 7-valent conjugate polysaccharide pneumococcal vaccine in the UK in 2002, it was hoped that invasive pneumococcal disease, including pleural empyemas in children would become a rarity, but this was found not to be the case, some of the persisting cases appearing to relate to an increased number of non-vaccine serotypes of pneumococcus. In 2010, a pneumococcal conjugate vaccine containing polysaccharide from thirteen common capsular types (PCV13) replaced PCV7, giving protection against against 6 additional serotypes (2).

Subdural empyema

Subdural empyema resulting from infection spreading from sinusitis is a recognised but fortunately rare complication seen in children, usually in the teenage years when their sinuses have developed as they reach adolescence. The route of infection to the subdural space is thought usually to be by the retrograde spread of infection from the nasal via the venous sinuses which are part of the venous system draining the brain. As a result of the absence of valves in these veins, infection can extend from a spreading thrombophlebitis not only into the subdural space, but can quickly extend to the cortical and subcortical veins of the brain itself. A thrombophlebitis once it takes hold can spread rapidly producing brain swelling. Because the dural space is an avascular space and empyema fluid collections are often of a similar density to surrounding brain substance, subdural empyemas can be difficult to visualise on a CT scan and are easier to visualise on a MRI scan. The important issue with a child presenting as Annie does is that the thrombophlebitis of the brain can develop very rapidly, leading to oedema and infarction of brain tissue with a rapid rise in intracranial pressure within a few hours and occasionally lead to cerebellar tonsillar herniation as in this case. Symptoms of this will include depressed conscious level and neck stiffness - mimicking meningitis, elevated blood pressure and slowed pulse rate - part of what is termed "Cushing's triad" of elevated systolic blood pressure (including widening pulse pressure), bradycardia and irregular breathing. The features in this case thus indicate a medical emergency requiring immediate neurosurgical intervention. Lumbar puncture on this child with neck stiffness would be likely to prove immediately fatal.

All the organisms listed above have the potential to produce a subdural empyema, and especially *Staph. aureus* and *Strep. pyogenes* can be associated with subdural empyema in children if the spread of infection comes from the ear, or following trauma. Anaerobic streptococci, in particular *Streptococcus anginosis* is associated in the majority of cases where infection has spread from a pansinusitis.

Tuberculosis

There has been a resurgence of tuberculosis in several parts of the world, including Eastern Europe, with frequently reported drug resistance to many first line drugs including rifampicin and isoniazid. The WHO estimated that world-wide, there were 9 million new cases of TB and 1.5 million died from the disease in 2013. It has been estimated that up to ⅓ of the world's population have latent TB. In the UK, most TB occurs in non-UK born individuals, living in large urban areas. The increasing population mobility combined with increasing drug resistance make contact tracing and microbial resistance studies very important. Local population screening for TB, and selective population immunisation with BCG are part of the UK policy of containment and hopefully eventual eradication of disease. Current population screening includes verbal screening, CXRs, tuberculin skin testing and interferon gamma release assays for latent tuberculous infection (2, 3).

Tuberculous meningitis is commonest in children under 6 years of age. It usually presents 3-6 months after initial infection and accompanies miliary TB in 50% of cases. There is often a 2-3 week history of irritability, anorexia and listlessness (1st stage disease) after which the disease passes into the 2nd stage where signs of specific cerebral involvement appear including raised intracranial pressure, nuchal rigidity, cranial nerve palsies and seizures. In the 3rd stage there is coma, rising fever, irregular breathing and pulse followed by death

Diagnosis of tuberculous meningitis should include a tuberculin skin test, radiographic studies for pulmonary and non-pulmonary TB (including miliary TB), careful examination of the fundi for miliary TB and for signs of papilloedema, and CSF examination if there is no contraindication to LP. The CSF will have a modest pleocytosis (mainly lymphocytes) with a rising CSF protein (depending on the stage of disease) and a falling CSF glucose (usually CSF to plasma glucose ratio <0.5). Mycobacteria should be carefully looked for with a ZN stained film on spun CSF samples and the CSF cultures specifically for TB. Treatment requires the advice of a specialist, and preferably with knowledge of any resistance pattern of the bacteria to anti-tuberculous drugs (4).

Statutory notification

The main purpose of the notification system is the detection and intervention in possible epidemics. It also enables surveillance data to be collected that can help in planning ways to prevent future outbreaks, but this is of secondary importance. The notifying doctor should complete a notification form immediately on diagnosis of a suspected notifiable disease. Only clinical suspicion of the disease is required, not laboratory confirmation, so the accuracy of diagnosis is not improved by the system.

Although many of the 32 diseases currently on the notification list are normally only to be found overseas, the list contains some infectious agents and specific diseases currently still potentially endemic in the UK such as invasive streptococcal disease and scarlet fever (5).

Syllabus Mapping

Infection, Immunology and Allergy

- Know about common infections of children in the UK and important worldwide infections, e.g. TB, HIV, hepatitis B, malaria, polio

- Know the UK national guidelines on notification of communicable diseases

- Know and understand the basic principles of infection control, how outbreaks of infection including nosocomial infection occur, and how they should be investigated

- Be able to assess and manage a febrile child and have knowledge of current evidence based guidelines

- Understand the principles and the rationale of immunisation programmes including the national immunisation programme for children in the UK

- Know when antimicrobials are indicated

- Understand the normal patterns and frequency of infections in childhood

Neurology

- Know the likely causes and management of meningitis/encephalitis and altered consciousness

Respiratory Medicine with ENT

- Know the causes and management of respiratory infection, earache, ear discharge, otitis media and glue ear

References

1. Ampofo K, Byington C. Management of parapneumonic empyema. The Pediatric infectious disease journal. 2007 May;26(5):445

2. Public Health England. Immunisation against infectious disease. https://www.gov.uk/government/collections/immunisation-against-infectious-disease-the-green-book

3. NICE. Tuberculosis NG33 January 2016 https://www.nice.org.uk/guidance/ng33

4. Török ME. Tuberculous meningitis: advances in diagnosis and treatment. British medical bulletin. 2015 Mar 1;113(1):117-31

5. Notifiable diseases and causative organisms: how to report. https://www.gov.uk/guidance/notifiable-diseases-and-causative-organisms-how-to-report

Further Reading

Ducel G, Fabry J, Nicolle L. Prevention of hospital acquired infections: a practical guide. Prevention of hospital acquired infections: a practical guide. 2002(Ed. 2)

Chapter 25: A pain in the back
Dr Beverley Almeida

Kate is a 13 year old girl who presents to the general paediatric clinic with a 6-month history of back pain. The pain is particularly in her lumbar spine and occurs throughout the day but is worse in the evening. She has tried simple analgesia such as paracetamol and ibuprofen but will little relief. She is feeling very anxious as this is now affecting her participation in gymnastics which she previously enjoyed. Her mother tells you that she seems to be "lopsided", her school skirt hem is higher on the left side with her left shoulder also being held higher than the right shoulder.

On examination her height and weight are both on the 91st centile. Her mother's height is on the 98th centile and she tells you that her father is also "very tall". She has shoulder asymmetry and pelvic tilt. There is an apparent curvature of the thoracic spine towards the left side with a more prominent left scapula which corrects on bending forwards. She has paraspinal muscle tenderness and spasm. She is able to bend forward and place her entire hand on the floor and you note that her wrists, elbows, knees and ankles all have an increased range of movement but none are swollen.

Q1. What is the most likely underlying cause of her back pain?

A. Enthesitis related arthritis
B. Hypermobility
C. Psychosomatic
D. Puberty related
E. Scoliosis

Q2. What is the scoliosis most likely due to?

A. Congenital spinal malformation
B. Ehlos Danlos syndrome
C. Idiopathic
D. Marfan's syndrome
E. Postural

Q3. Which one of the following specialists should you refer this child to next?

A. Chronic pain services
B. Geneticist
C. Physiotherapist
D. Rheumatologist
E. Spinal surgeon

Answers and Rationale

Q1. **B: Hypermobility**
Q2. **E: Postural**
Q3. **C: Physiotherapist**

Kate has two coexisting conditions, namely hypermobility and scoliosis. They are not necessarily associated with each other, but you should remain open that any patient can have more than one diagnosis; in particular many patients with juvenile idiopathic arthritis can also have hypermobility.

Hypermobility

Many children are hypermobile. It is a normal variant up until the age of 5 to 8 years old. However in some children it can persist and can be used to the individual's advantage, such as making them successful ballet dancers, gymnasts or contortionists and not cause them any them whatsoever.

In hypermobility the range of movement of certain or all joints is increased beyond normal and in some children, if the muscles supporting those joints are not strong, pain can ensue (1). Pain that worsens during the course of the day after activity is usually non-inflammatory in nature (inflammatory pain usually improves after activity, with gelling occurring after rest periods). Hypermobility of the spine can lead to back pain if the paraspinal muscles are weak and if core stability is poor (2). In these cases if physiotherapy is not instituted early, children can develop problems with mobility and are sometimes incorrectly are managed with escalation of pain medications and the use of crutches and wheelchairs. In children most cases of scoliosis do not cause pain, this would be a red flag and may indicate an underlying malignancy. There is nothing in Kate's history to suggest a bone tumour, where the pain is characteristically at night.

It is important to examine the joints carefully and obtain a feel for if the joints move beyond the range of movement. The Beighton score was validated in adults and although can be used in children, it only tests certain joints (with a total score of 9, 1 each the left and right sides and 1 for the spine):

- the thumb MCP which can be placed on the forearm
- the fingers moving greater than 90 degrees of flexion
- the elbows moving greater than 180 degrees of extension
- the knees moving greater than 180 degrees of extension and
- lumbar spine flexion so that the entire palm of the hand can be placed on the floor

You need to score more than 4 to be said to have generalised hypermobility, but it is possible to have only a few localised hypermobile joints. A physiotherapy assessment can formally measure the range of movement.

The vast majority of hypermobility seen in general paediatric clinics is totally benign and if there are no symptoms of pain or decreased mobility require no further investigation and tests are nor usually warranted.

Only a very small number of patients have Marfan's or Ehlers Danlos syndrome and these diagnoses are usually quite striking on examination. Children with Marfan's syndrome will be tall with archynodactyly, pectus excavatum, a high arched palate and be myopic. In these children cardiac review with echocardiography and an ophthalmology assessment are necessary. In Ehlers Danlos Syndrome there will be hyperextinsibility of the skin, poor wound healing and sometimes blue sclera. There is an increased risk of aortic regurgitation and dissection of the aorta so referral to cardiology is again indicated. As both conditions are autosomal dominant there is likely to be a family history and geneticist referral and services would be warranted.

In Kate's case the best next step would be referral to physiotherapy services to help improve muscle strength (3), which would thereby decrease the pain from the hypermobile joints and would also help the scoliosis. In simple hypermobility causing pain, physiotherapy is the best first line management with psychological support and occupational therapy input.

Scoliosis

Children with hypermobility tend to have poor posture due to their lack of core stability and hence often slouch or fidget to remain comfortable. The scoliosis in this case is therefore most likely non-structural, or postural.

Scoliosis can occur during growth in puberty, but there is no mention of this in the history and again there are no features that indicate a chronic infection, inflammatory cause or malignancy. The lopsided skirt hem and her left shoulder being higher than the other is commonly seen due to carrying a heavy schoolbag on one shoulder on a daily basis (2) (fashion conscious teenage girls do not like to wear backpacks with a strap on each shoulder!). This in itself is very bad for posture and can consequently cause a pelvic tilt.

Asymmetrical trunk skin creases may also be noted and the correction of the scoliosis on bending forwards fits with there being a non-structural cause rather than a structural one where the scoliosis remains.

Imaging can be helpful to assess the scoliosis. First line imaging is spinal anteriorposterior (AP) and lateral x-rays before an MRI. MRI would be considered first line in the case of red flags or painful scoliosis. Pulmonary functions tests may also be necessary in the instance of a severe thoracic scoliosis.

In Kate's case, physiotherapy would also benefit the scoliosis too. If scoliosis is structural then referral to a dedicated spinal team is necessary and treatment would include physiotherapy, spinal bracing or surgery depending on severity.

Scoliosis can also be seen in neuromuscular disorders such as muscular dystrophies, cerebral palsy and also in neurofibromatosis. In children scoliosis rarely causes pain, but if present, or if there are associated neurological signs, these would be considered red flags and a spinal tumour should be ruled out.

Enthesitis Related Arthritis (ERA)

ERA is a sub group of Juvenile Idiopathic Arthritis, typically seen in boys over the age of 10 who may or may not be HLA B27 positive. Symptoms include long-term lower back, hip and buttock pain whilst walking (sacroiliac joint involvement). Examination findings include tenderness on palpation of the sacroiliac joints and tenderness on palpation over tendons such as the Achilles tendon.

Back pain

Back pain is a common symptom in adolescents. It is much more unusual in younger children and toddlers who are not able to accurately localize where pain originates from. In this younger age group, a low threshold for imaging with an MRI and urinary catecholamines and catecholamine metabolites is needed to rule out a spinal or bone tumour or neuroblastoma.

Chronic non-specific lower back pain in older children and adolescents is more likely due to posture, carrying heavy schoolbags and lack of physical activity. For this, physiotherapy is very helpful. If there are no red flags then imaging is not needed. If indicated MRI, CT and bone scans are usually more helpful than simple x-rays for identifying any of the organic pathologies listed below.

Other musculoskeletal conditions causing back pain include:

- Hypermobility
- Biomechanical
- Chronic pain
- Spondylosis
- Inflammatory arthritis in particular ERA
- Disc degeneration
- Tumours
- Osteoporosis

Syllabus Mapping

Musculoskeletal

- Know about the assessment, causes and initial management of joint laxity and joint swelling

- Know the causes of back pain and initial management

- Know how to recognise the various causes of scoliosis and how they present

References

1. Kemp S1, Roberts I, Gamble C, Wilkinson S, Davidson JE, Baildam EM, Cleary AG, McCann LJ, Beresford MW. A randomized comparative trial of generalized vs targeted physiotherapy in the management of childhood hypermobility. Rheumatology. 2010 Feb;49(2):315-25

2. Rodríguez-Oviedo P, Ruano-Ravina A, Pérez-Ríos M, García FB, Gómez-Fernández D, Fernández-Alonso A, Carreira-Núñez I, García-Pacios P, Turiso J. School children's backpacks, back pain and back pathologies. Archives of disease in childhood. 2012 Aug 1;97(8):730-2

3. Armon K. Musculoskeletal pain and hypermobility in children and young people: is it benign joint hypermobility syndrome?. Archives of disease in childhood. 2015 Jan 1;100(1):2-3

Further Reading

Foster HE, Brogan PA. Paediatric Rheumatology. Oxford University Press; 2012 Jun 14

Chapter 26: A busy advice line
Dr Jim Gould

26

You have rotated to an ST2 post in infectious diseases. On your first morning you receive several phone calls requesting advice. A GP calls you about a 2 year old girl from eastern Africa who has recently arrived with her mother in the UK as a refugee. Both the child and her mother are infected with HIV. The child is clinically well, her CD4 count is not suppressed and she is not at present on anti-retroviral therapy. The child has no history of being immunised.

Q1. Which one of the following immunisations is contraindicated?

A.   BCG
B.   Hepatitis B
C.   Influenza A
D.   MMR
E.   Varicella

A 4 year old boy with acute lymphoblastic leukaemia has recently been admitted to the oncology ward for further chemotherapy. The oncology team want to know if he should be considered for passive antibody protection following a recent exposure.

Q2. Which one of the following viral infections is passive antibody protection advised?

A.   Hepatitis B
B.   Infectious mononucleosis
C.   Influenza A
D.   Measles
E.   Rubella

A GP calls about an 18 month old boy who has received no immunisations. His mother has been reluctant to agree to him being immunised because of possible adverse effects to immunisation.

Q3. Which one of the following would be a contraindication to the child's immunisation?

A.   Evolving neurological condition with possible regression
B.   Family history of adverse reaction following immunisation
C.   History in the child of epilepsy
D.   Sibling with epilepsy
E.   Sibling with immune suppression following chemotherapy for leukaemia

Answers and Rationale

Q1   A: BCG
Q2   D: Measles
Q3   A: Evolving neurological condition with possible regression

Live vaccines can sometimes cause severe or fatal infections in immunosuppressed individuals because of uncontrolled systemic replication of the vaccine strain. It is for this reason that live vaccines should generally be avoided in severely immune suppressed children, such as:

- Severe immune deficiency, such as SCID and Wiskott-Aldrich syndrome
- Children undergoing chemotherapy or radiotherapy for malignant disease, or those who have finished treatment within the last 6 months
- Children who have received a solid organ transplant currently on immune suppressive therapy.
- Children who have received a bone marrow transplant until at least 12 months after stopping immune suppressive therapy
- Children on high dose systemic steroids
- Children on immune suppressive therapy for other diseases
- Children with HIV and severe immune suppression as judged by CD4 count

Live vaccines in current or recent use in the UK:
Bacterial:
- BCG

Viral:
- Measles
- Mumps
- Rubella
- Rotavirus
- Influenza*
- Oral Polio (OPV)$
- Varicella
- Yellow Fever

In a child with HIV and a normal CD4 count, BCG and Yellow Fever are the only contraindicated vaccines. There have been reports of dissemination of BCG in HIV positive individuals, and from infants immunised who are in contact with HIV positive mothers with immune suppression. In a child susceptible to varicella and normal CD4, varicella vaccine is indicated to reduce the risk of serious varicella or zoster later if their clinical condition deteriorates. Similarly MMR and Rotavirus vaccines can be safely given and OPV is no longer routinely available in the UK.

- *All but one Influenza vaccine is inactivated, and all but one of these are administered intramuscularly. The exception is the live vaccine (Fluenz Tetra®) which is administered by nasal spray. Most of the vaccines are prepared from viruses grown in embryonated hens eggs
- $OPV is no longer available for routine use and will only be available for outbreak control. OPV contains live attenuated strains of poliomyelitis virus types 1, 2 and 3 grown in cultures of monkey kidney cells or in human diploid (MRC-5) cells.

Passive antibody protection refers to the process of providing IgG antibodies to protect against infection. It provides immediate, but short-lived protection (several weeks up to 4 months). Passive immunity can occur naturally, for example when maternal IgG antibodies are transferred to the fetus through the placenta or be acquired when at risk individuals receive antibodies to a defined infection These antibodies are produced by obtaining serum from immune individuals, pooling this and then concentrating the immunoglobulin fraction.

Passive antibody protection is considered in the following situations:

a. Protection against tetanus with human tetanus immunoglobulin, where there is significant risk of infection from a penetrating wound and active tetanus immunisation has not occurred, is incomplete or when there is a very high risk of infection.

b. Zoster immune globulin (VZIG) for protection of varicella non-immune immunosuppressed children post varicella exposure.

c. Human immunoglobulin post exposure to measles in a measles non-immune immunosuppressed child at risk.

d. Palivizumab (Synagis) for the prevention of serious lower respiratory tract disease requiring hospitalisation caused by respiratory syncytial virus (RSV) in children at high risk for RSV disease. These include ex-preterm infants with chronic lung disease, infants with other respiratory diseases who remain in oxygen at the start of the RSV season, haemodynamically significant congenital heart disease and children with SCID. It is also indicated in some ex-preterm infants without significant respiratory disease depending upon their gestational age at birth and chronological age at the start of the bronchiolitis season (see chapter 27 "Green Book" (1))

e. Hepatitis B immunoglobulin (HBIG) is given after exposure to hepatitis B-infected blood to provide rapid protection until hepatitis B vaccine, which should be given at the same time, becomes effective.

Herd protection of the un-immunised occurs when a significant proportion of the population is immune. The WHO's target to establish herd immunity is for 95% of children to be immunised. Several vaccine scares in the late 1990's and early 21st century led to decreased uptake of vaccines with immunisation rates below that required for herd immunity. There are very few occasions when deferral of active immunisation is required. Minor illnesses without fever or systemic upset are not valid reasons to postpone immunisation. If an individual is acutely unwell, immunisation may be postponed until they have fully recovered. This is to avoid wrongly attributing any new symptom or the progression of symptoms to the vaccine. In children who present without having had routine immunisation, and where there is reluctance on the part of the parent to agree to immunisation, every effort should be made to reassure and inform the parent to allow permission for immunisation to take place. Other than a history of anaphylaxis to a previous vaccine, or an unwell child with a fever, a child with an evolving neurological condition which may be leading to developmental regression is the only reason for deferment of immunisation, until the neurological condition has resolved or stabilised. A history of epilepsy in the child or a sibling, a sibling with immune suppression and a family history of adverse reaction to immunisation are NOT contraindications to immunisation of that child (1).

Infection control

Two basic principles govern the main measures that should be taken in order to prevent the spread of nosocomial infections in hospitals or health-care facilities: (i) separate the infection source from the rest of the hospital and (ii) cut off any route of transmission. The separation of the source includes not only the isolation of infected patients but also all "aseptic techniques" — the measures that are intended to act as a barrier between infected or potentially contaminated tissue and the environment, including other patients and hospital personnel.

Microorganisms can be transmitted from their source to a new host through direct or indirect contact, in the air, or by vectors. Vector-borne transmission is typical of countries in which insects, arthropods, and other parasites are widespread. Airborne transmission occurs only with microorganisms that are dispersed into the air and can infect another patient with a minimal infective dose. Only a few bacteria and viruses are present in expired air, and these are dispersed in large numbers only as a result of sneezing or coughing. Direct contact between patients does not usually occur in health-care facilities, but an infected health-care worker can touch a patient and directly transmit a large number of microorganisms to the new host. The most frequent route of transmission is indirect contact. The infected patient touches, and contaminates an object, an instrument, or a surface. Subsequent contact between that item and another patient contaminates the second individual who may then develop an infection. During general care and/or medical treatment the hands of health-care workers often come into close contact with patients. The hands of the clinical personnel are thus the most frequent vehicles for nosocomial infections. Transmission by this route is much more common than vector-borne or air-borne transmission or other forms of direct or indirect contact (3).

Syllabus Mapping

Infection, Immunology and Allergy

- Know about common infections of children in the UK and important worldwide infections, e.g. TB, HIV, hepatitis B, malaria, polio

- Know and understand the basic principles of infection control, how outbreaks of infection including nosocomial infection occur, and how they should be investigated

- Understand the principles and the rationale of immunisation programmes including the national immunisation programme for children in the UK

- Know and understand the indications, contraindications, complications and controversies of routine childhood immunisations and be able to advise parents about immunisations

Patient Safety and Clinical Governance

- Know the main routes of transmission of hospital acquired infections and their prevention

References and Further Reading

1. Public Health England. Immunisation against infectious disease. https://www.gov.uk/government/collections/immunisation-against-infectious-disease-the-green-book

2. Baxter D. Active and passive immunity, vaccine types, excipients and licensing. Occupational Medicine. 2007 Dec 1;57(8):552-6

3. Ducel G, Fabry J, Nicolle L. Prevention of hospital acquired infections: a practical guide. 2002(Ed. 2)

Chapter 27: Asthma Clinic
Dr Bijan Shahrad and Dr Arvind Shah

(27)

You are seeing patients in the asthma clinic.

This is a list of investigations:

A. Blood sample for genetic test
B. Bronchoscopy
C. Cilia motility study
D. CT scan of the thorax
E. Diary of Peak Flow measurements

F. Oesophageal pH study
G. Spirometery
H. Sputum sample
I. Sweat test
J. Sleep study

For each of the following children select the most appropriate investigation:

Q1a. Arran is a 2 year old boy who has a recurrent chesty cough, which has not improved with inhaled salbutamol and inhaled steroids. His mother says he has haemorrhoids. His weight is on the 10th centile. His chest x-ray is reported as being normal.

Q1b. Beth is a 6 year old girl who is woken frequently at night by a cough. She also coughs when running about. Her cough is improved by inhaled salbutamol via a large volume spacer. Her weight is on the 50th centile. Her chest x-ray is reported as normal.

Q1c. Charles a 2 year old boy presents with abrupt onset of cough. The cough started after he had been at a birthday party a week ago. Another child at the party has subsequently been diagnosed with chicken pox. His weight is on the 50th centile. There is a wheeze heard at the right mid zone. His chest x-ray is reported as normal.

Dan is a 4 year old boy with Down's syndrome. He has asthma which is well controlled on inhaled salbutamol. His mother is concerned that he appears tired almost every day. He seems to sleep well but snores at night.

Q2. Which of the following is the most important next management step?

A. Commence steroid inhalers
B. Diary of Peak Flow measurements
C. Otoscopy
D. Referral for ENT examination
E. Sleep study

Answers and Rationale

Q1a.   I: Sweat test
Q1b.   E: Diary of Peak Flow measurements
Q1c.   B: Bronchoscopy
Q2.   E: Sleep Study

This chapter identifies a common issue in paediatrics and medicine in general. People are frequently "labelled" as having a common diagnosis, in this case "Asthma", when in fact they may have a different underlying aetiology for their symptoms. When approaching any clinical presentation styled question it is important to identify any concerning or unusual elements of the history. For the first boy Arran, the fact that the cough is 'chesty' and that he is failing to thrive coupled with the history of haemorrhoids should start alarm bells ringing that he may have Cystic Fibrosis (CF).

CF is a multisystem, autosomal recessive disorder and the most common life threatening genetic disorder in Caucasian population. Inherited as an autosomal recessive condition, 1 in 25 Caucasian's are carriers with deltaF508 being the most common mutation (66-70% of known cases of CF). Caused by the presence of a mutation in both copies of the gene for cystic fibrosis trans-membrane conductor regulator (CFTR), it can present early as meconium ileus in new born babies, or later as failure to thrive (due to pancreatic involvement) or recurrent chest infections (1). To answer the question, knowledge of diagnostic tests for CF is needed – as the stem asks for the 'best next step'. This is important as some of the options are used for the management of CF but not as a diagnostic tool. A sweat test is the gold standard diagnostic test for CF. It works by applying pilocarpine along with a small electrical stimulation to a small area of skin to encourage sweat formation and measuring the amount of chloride in the sweat. If the sweat chloride is less than 40mmol/l it is a negative test, if 40-60mmol then it is a borderline test. If the chloride concentration is greater or equal to 60mmol/L then this indicates for CF. A positive sweat test can also occur in children receiving topiramate, underweight infants, Addison's disease, nephrogenic diabetes insipidus, hypothyroidism and if the sweat site has active eczema though these conditions should be distinguished from CF by the presenting phenotype.

There are more than 1,000 different alterations of the CF gene. The standard genetic analyses will detect approximately 90% of these mutations with the rarer mutations not tested for. Therefore if the genetic test is not homozygous for the a CF gene defect it may be that the individual carries one of these rarer mutations and does indeed have CF. For this reason genetic testing should not be the first line test for CF. In preterm infants and those less than 2 weeks of age genetic testing is often the first line investigation as they often do not produce a sufficient volume of sweat to be analysed (2).

Cystic Fibrosis is a multi-organ disease (see table 27.1). In the lungs the mucus clogs the airways and traps bacteria leading to recurrent infections and excessive lung damage (bronchiectasis) and eventually respiratory failure. *Staphlococcus aures*, *Haemophilus influenza* and *Pseudomonas aeruginosa* are the most prevalent infections in CF (3). Cardiorespiratory complications are the most common cause of death.

CT scans can be used to allow assessment of the evolution of CF disease but is not a diagnostic tool. Bronchoscopy is also a useful tool in CF to obtain lower airways specimens from children who are not able to expectorate. It can be used therefore to guide antibiotic treatment, Pancreatic involvement can cause CF related diabetes (CFRD) and is seen in 30% of adult patients. Exocrine pancreatic insufficiency is common and can present as fatty, bulky stools due to malabsorption and failure to thrive (as in this case). Enzyme replacement is the main stay of treatment (Creon). Constipation occurs due to altered intestinal fluid composition, which can lead to haemorrhoids.

Organ System	Complication	Treatment	Long term complication
Lung	Mucus build up Impaired ciliary clearance. Inflammation + infection.	Prophylactic antibiotics. Methods of exportation (physiotherapy, nebulisers). Intravenous antibiotics for exacerbations.	Bronchiectasis. Pulmonary hypertension. Cardiorespiratory failure.
Pancreas (Exocrine)	Pancreatic insufficiency. Steatorrhoea Malabsorption. A,D,E + K vitamin deficiency. Coagulation disorders.	Supplemental pancreatic enzymes (Creon). Dietician involvement. Gastrostomy in severely affected.	Failure to thrive.
Pancreas (Endocrine)	Islet cell damage Cystic Fibrosis related diabetes. Vitamin D deficiency.	Insulin. Vitamin D supplementation.	CFRD. Reduced bone mineral density.
ENT	Polyp formation	Surgery	Blockage of nasal passage
GI	Meconium ileus (neonate). Rectal prolapse. Haemorrhoids. GORD. Distal intestinal obstruction syndrome. Cirrhosis.	Stool softeners. Anti-reflux medication. Surgery.	Bleeding disorders. Bowel obstruction. Adhesions.
Reproductive	Congenital absence vas deferens. Poor motility. Thickened cervical mucus,	IVF	

Table 27.1: Systemic involvement of CF

With Beth's presentation, the presence of eczema and response to β^2 agonists means it is likely that she does indeed have asthma. Troublesome night time symptoms indicate the likely need for escalation in her treatment with the addition of inhaled corticosteroids. Monitoring peak flow will allow you to have an objective measure of the response to inhaled corticosteorids. Please see chapter 10 and 28 for further information on the management of asthma.

When Charles presents with an abrupt onset of a cough, you should consider a diagnosis of an inhaled foreign body. Being at a birthday party increases the risk of finding objects to inhale. Children develop chicken pox all the time so that wouldn't be unusual in any history.

Additionally, the incubation period for varicella is 7 – 21 days with varicella pneumonia presenting after the onset of rash. Being told the wheeze is confined to right mid zone makes viral induced wheeze (classically diffuse wheeze) unlikely and a foreign body more likely due to classical right main bronchus preference. The fact the Chest x-ray is normal is put there to cause doubt, but it may be normal in up to 35% of cases of foreign body inhalation (4). Changes are best seen on inspiratory films, which are difficult in uncooperative children. Bronchoscopy is the investigation of choice to both identify and remove the foreign body and will require referral to ENT or tertiary respiratory specialists. Urgent bronchoscopy is essential as the area of lung being under ventilated remains well perfused, causing a V/Q mismatch and thus bronchiectasis. A CT scan of thorax would aid in the diagnosis of a foreign body but would not help with the management of removal and so is incorrect.

Dan's presentation is classical of obstructive sleep apnoea (OSA). This is caused by a significant obstruction of the upper airways during sleep, resulting in apnoea (complete cessation of airflow), hypopnoea (significantly reduced airflow passage), hypoventilation, hypercapnea and hypoxemia. OSA is one of the common presentation of children with large adenoids and tonsils. Children with Down's syndrome are at increased risk (30-60%) due to factors including adenotonsillar hyperplasia, midfacial and mandibular hypoplasia, hypotonia, small upper airways and macroglossia (5). The investigation of choice would be a sleep study, which would guide treatment

Syllabus Mapping

Respiratory Medicine with ENT

- Know the presentations of cystic fibrosis and the principles of treatment

- Understand the causes of chronic cough and appropriate investigations

References and Further Reading

1. Marcdante SJ, Kliegman RM, Jenson HB, Behrman RE. 6th ed. Canada: Saunders Elsevier; 2011. Nelson Essential of Pediatrics; pgs.521-522

2. Heap S. Guidelines for the Performance of the Sweat Test for the Investigation of Cystic Fibrosis in the UK ver 2. 2009

3. Shields M D, O'Connor, Respiratory Paediatrics chapter in MRCPCH Master course, Royal College of Paediatrics and Child Health: Elsevier, 2008: 252-256

4. Cevik M, Gokdemir MT, Boleken ME, Sogut O, Kurkcuoglu C. The characteristics and outcomes of foreign body ingestion and aspiration in children due to lodged foreign body in the aerodigestive tract. Pediatric Emergency Care. 2013 Jan 1;29(1):53-7

5. Alida Goffinski, Maria A. Stanley, Nichole Shephered, Nichole Duvall, Sandra B. Jenkinson, Charlene Davis, Marilyn J. Bull. Obstructive sleep apnea in young infants with Downs syndrome evaluated in a Down's syndrome specialty clinic. American Journal of Medical Genetics. 2015 Jan 167 (2): 324-330

Chapter 28: A Wheezy day
Dr Arvind Shah and Dr Emily Isaacs

(28)

You are on-call for paediatric admissions. Eric, a 9 year old boy with a long standing history of asthma attends with an acute exacerbation of breathlessness with wheeze. On admission his oxygen saturations were 91% in air and his heart rate was 120/minute. He had widespread wheeze and was using his accessory muscles. The emergency department ST1 doctor gave him nebulised salbutamol and ipratropium bromide driven by oxygen and oral prednisolone. After this his oxygen saturations are 92% in 50% oxygen but he is drowsy with poor respiratory effort. He calls you asking for advice and you arrange to review him with your consultant.

Q1. Which one treatment should you advise the ST1 doctor to initiate whilst you are on your way to review Eric?

A.   Intravenous bolus of hydrocortisone
B.   Intravenous bolus of magnesium
C.   Intravenous bolus of salbutamol
D.   Intravenous magnesium infusion
E.   Intravenous aminophylline infusion

After reviewing Eric, the emergency department doctor asks you to review 3 more children.

This is a list of medications available in the emergency department:

A.   Inhaled ipratropium via spacer
B.   Inhaled salbutamol via spacer
C.   Intravenous aminophylline
D.   Intravenous hydrocortisone
E.   Intravenous magnesium sulphate

F.   Intravenous salbutamol
G.   Nebulised adrenaline driven by oxygen
H.   Nebulised salbutamol driven by oxygen
I.   Oral prednisolone
J.   Oxygen

Which is most appropriate initial medication for the each of the following children presenting to the emergency department?

Q2a. A 3 year old girl with a history of asthma attends with an acute exacerbation and has oxygen saturations of 90% in air. She has widespread wheeze on auscultation.

Q2b. A 5 year old boy presents with a cough and has oxygen saturations of 96% in air. He has widespread wheeze on auscultation

Q2c. A 6 month old boy with acute respiratory distress has oxygen saturations of 90% in air. He has widespread wheeze and crackles on auscultation.

Answers and Rationale

Q1. **C: Intravenous bolus of salbutamol**
Q2. **H: Nebulised salbutamol driven by oxygen**
Q3. **B: Inhaled salbutamol via spacer**
Q4. **J: Oxygen**

In the first case this child is initially presenting with a severe exacerbation of his asthma which despite initial appropriate management has demonstrated deterioration with him becoming drowsy and his respiratory effort deteriorating and having "life threatening asthma" (see Table 28.1). In this situation urgent review by a senior clinician is required and a consideration of intensive care admission is required.

Severe Asthma	Life Threatening Asthma
• breathlessness preventing talking in full sentences or feeding • SpO2 <92% PEF 33-50% best or predicted • tachycardia (heart rate >125 (>5 years) or >140 (2-5 years)) • tachypnea (>30 breaths/min (>5 years) or >40 (2-5 years)).	• oxygen saturations < 92% in air • peak expiratory flow less than <33% best or predicted • silent chest • cyanosis • poor respiratory effort • hypotension • exhaustion • confusion

Table 28.1: Clinical features of severe and life threatening asthma in children > 2 years (1)

It is important that you are familiar with the latest guidance on management of acute severe and life threatening asthma. The SIGN guidelines (Scottish Intercollegiate Guidelines Network), states that if there is failure to respond to inhaled therapy then a bolus of intravenous salbutamol should be administered (1) (see table 28.2). It is also important that you monitor the response to any treatment carefully with the following parameters (1);

- Pulse rate – increasing tachycardia generally denotes worsening asthma; a fall in heart rate in life threatening asthma is a pre-terminal event
- Respiratory rate and degree of breathlessness
- Use of accessory muscles of respiration – best noted by palpation of neck muscles
- Amount of wheezing – which might become biphasic or less apparent with increasing airways obstruction
- Degree of agitation and conscious level – always give calm reassurance

It is important to note however that clinical signs correlate poorly with the severity of airways obstruction and some children with acute severe asthma do not appear distressed.

Oxygen therapy	• Saturations should be maintained at 94% and above.
Bronchodilators	• Mild-moderate asthma: Metered dose inhaler and spacer to administer bronchodilator therapy. • Add ipratropium bromide to nebulised beta-2 agonist therapy if symptoms do not resolve with initial treatment.
Steroids	• Give early to maximize effect. 3 day course, not tapered unless more than 14 days have been administered. • Prednisolone; < 2 years: 10 mg, 2-5 years: 20 mg, >5 years: 30-40mg prednisolone. • Consider intravenous (IV) steroids if repeatedly vomiting oral steroid.
Second line treatment	• IV salbutamol bolus in severe asthma if not responding to inhaled treatment. • IV aminophylline in unresponsive severe or life-threatening asthma. • IV magnesium sulphate does not yet have an established evidence base but is a "safe treatment".

Table 28.2: SIGN management of acute asthma (1)

The next two children (Q2a and 2b) also have acute wheeze but are presenting with milder symptoms. The first child has low oxygen saturations so requires oxygen as well as bronchodilator therapy. The second child has normal oxygen saturations but widespread wheeze. There is now good evidence that inhaled β2 agonists from a metered dose inhaler are effective and are the preferred method of administration for mild to moderate asthma exacerbations.

The 6 month old child is presenting with the commonest causes of wheeze in children, bronchiolitis. Bronchiolitis is a lower respiratory tract infection, most commonly caused by the respiratory syncitial virus (RSV) and generally affects infants under the age of 1 year. It typically presents with a cough, wheeze, and breathlessness occurring over several days. Widespread crackles and/or wheeze are typical findings on auscultation. The breathlessness may persist for several days and commonly the airways remain hyper-reactive for several weeks, leading to recurrent cough and wheeze.

There is no effective treatment for bronchiolitis with the management being mainly supportive. Salbutamol therapy is ineffective as children of this age do not have effective beta-2 adrenoreceptors in their lungs. In patients with bronchiolitis, oxygen saturations should be maintained at 92% or above, with the use of oxygen. Children with severe respiratory distress will require additional supportive therapy which may include nasogastric fluids or intravenous fluids. If respiratory failure is evolving. CPAP (continuous positive airway pressure) or ventilation may be needed for respiratory support (2). Certain high risk groups of children receive passive immunisation against bronchiolitis as it has been demonstrated to reduce the severity of respiratory symptoms and the incidence of intensive care admission in those groups (3). This is discussed in chapter 26.

Syllabus Mapping

Respiratory Medicine with ENT

- Know how to assess and manage children with acute asthma and wheeze and plan long term management

- Understand the causes of chronic cough and appropriate investigations

References and Further Reading

1. British Thoracic Society Scottish Intercollegiate Guidelines Network. British guideline on the management of asthma. Thorax. 2014 Nov 1;69(Suppl 1):i1-92

2. NICE Guideline: bronchiolitis in children. (NG9) Archives of disease in childhood-Education & practice edition. 2015 Dec 1:edpract-2015

3. Andabaka T, Nickerson JW, Rojas-Reyes M, Rueda J, Bacic Vrca V, Barsic B. Monoclonal antibody for reducing the risk of respiratory syncytial virus infection in children. Cochrane Database of Systematic Reviews 2013, Issue 4. Art. No.: CD006602

Chapter 29: A Sleepy baby
Dr James Davison and Dr Maureen Cleary

(29)

Irfan, a 7 day old baby boy is referred to you by the ST1 doctor in the emergency department. He has been vomiting all of his feeds for the past 24 hours and is sleepy. He was born at term by normal delivery 72 hours after rupture of membranes with a birth weight of 2.7 kg. He is the second child to his parents who are second cousins. He was discharged home on day 2 and seen by the midwife on day 5 for a routine visit when he appeared well and was establishing breast feeds.

Blood results are as follows:

Glucose	1.8mmol/l
C-reactive protein	<1mg/l
Ammonia	347 umol/l
Haemoglobin	145g/l
Platelet	308x10^9/l
White cell count	5.6x10^9/l

Blood gas:

pH	7.20
pCO$_2$	3.5 kPa
Bicarbonate	12 mmol/l
Base excess	-14

An intravenous cannula has been sited and antibiotics have been administered.

On examination he is very quiet and poorly responsive. His temperature is 36.4°C respiratory rate is 72/minute, oxygen saturations 98% in air, heart rate 150/minute and central capillary refill less than 2 seconds. He weighs 2.5 kg. He has no intercostal recessions. His chest is clear and heart sounds are normal. He is mildly jaundiced and his liver is just palpable below the right costal margin. His anterior fontanelle is full.

Q1. What factor in the history and examination is most suggestive of an inherited metabolic disorder?

A. Palpable liver edge
B. Parental consanguinity
C. Pattern of onset of symptoms
D. Poorly responsive on examination
E. Tachycardia and tachypnoea

Q2. What is the most likely metabolic diagnosis?

A. An organic aciduria
B. Glycogen storage disease
C. Homocystinuria
D. Mucopolysaccharidosis (Hurler syndrome)
E. Phenylketonuria (PKU)

The metabolic laboratory calls to report an abnormal result from the day 5 newborn screening.

Q3. What is the most likely diagnosis in keeping with the presentation?

A. Glutaric aciduria type 1
B. Homocystinuria
C. Isovaleric acidaemia
D. Mucopolysaccharidosis
E. Phenylketonuria

Answers and Rationale

Q1. **C: Pattern of onset of symptoms**
Q2. **A: An organic aciduria**
Q3. **C: Isovaleric acidaemia**

Inherited metabolic disorders (IMDs) are each individually rare, but together affect up to 900 children born each year in the UK. They are caused by deficient activity of individual enzymes, resulting in disturbed function of many different metabolic pathways. IMDs can present with acute biochemical disturbances, with dysfunction of any organ system, and at any age ranging from early neonatal and even *in utero* presentations to later more slowly progressive disorders. Good history taking, careful examination, judicious use of biochemical tests, and awareness of modes of presentation are key to making the diagnosis and instigating what can be life-saving treatment.

Neonates with IMD are usually well at birth with no physical signs, and *in utero* babies are protected by the placento-maternal circulation which effectively continuously dialyses out any metabolic toxins. The catabolic stress of birth coupled with disconnection from the placenta and the introduction of a substantial protein load through milk feeds can lead to deranged metabolism. Babies typically present after an initial period of appearing well, but can become progressively unwell with vomiting, lethargy, seizures leading to coma as different toxins accumulate. Toxins include organic acids, ammonia, lactic acid, associated with metabolic acidosis and hypoglycaemia.

The clinical presentation is often indistinguishable from sepsis, or duct-dependent cardiac lesions, and all of these possibilities should be considered in parallel in the unwell neonate. Indeed, as in this case, there may be risk factors for sepsis (prolonged rupture of membranes) as well as pointers to metabolic disease. Parental consanguinity and detailed family history are important to establish as most IMD are inherited in an autosomal recessive manner, however IMD still occur in the offspring of unrelated parents.

The initial assessment of the collapsed/unwell infant should proceed according to standard resuscitation guidelines, evaluating Airway, Breathing and Circulation. Blood glucose should always be checked, and the finding of hypoglycaemia should prompt swift intervention to correct the low blood glucose, ideally after collection of an aliquot of blood for a "hypoglycaemia screen" although the priority is to treat the hypoglycaemia. In any unwell neonate with abnormal neurological findings it is imperative to check the basic metabolic parameters including glucose, blood gas, lactate, ketones (urine dipstick or bedside blood monitor) and ammonia.

The finding of abnormal results on this initial panel of investigations should prompt discussion with a Metabolic Specialist and consideration of focussed further biochemical investigations in parallel with initiation of emergency management. Hyperammonaemia is seen in the urea cycle disorders, but is also a feature of the organic acid disorders where there is secondary inhibition of the urea cycle. Ammonia is extremely neurotoxic, and requires prompt treatment. Elevated ketones in a neonate is abnormal, and this finding is strongly suggestive of an organic acid disorder especially if there is also metabolic acidosis with a raised anion gap. Strongly elevated ketones in an infant with suppressed neurological status or seizures but with normal blood gas and ammonia is seen in Maple Syrup Urine Disease. Deranged liver function tests are seen in infants with galactosaemia, tyrosinaemia and the fatty acid oxidation defects, the most common of which is medium chain acyl-CoA dehydrogenase deficiency (MCADD).

The biochemical findings in the case described here show a severe metabolic acidosis, hypoglycaemia and hyperammonaemia. Further investigations would show elevated ketones, and the calculated anion gap demonstrates this to be significantly elevated. A metabolic acidosis with an elevated anion gap (calculated as $[Na^+ + K^+] - [Cl^- + HCO3^-]$, normal 8-17mmol/l) implies there is accumulation of an acid (such as an organic acid or lactate) that is donating hydrogen ions (H^+); a metabolic acidosis with a normal anion gap implies that the low pH is caused by loss of bicarbonate either through the kidneys (e.g. renal Fanconi syndrome) or the gastrointestinal tract (e.g. diarrhoeal illness). Ketones are usually not detected in neonates even when unwell unless there is a metabolic disorder. The organic acids that accumulate are toxic and inhibit normal gluconeogenesis, and this together with the catabolism of ketogenic amino acids drives the excessive production of ketone bodies. This biochemical picture, together with the elevated ammonia, points towards an organic aciduria as the most likely metabolic diagnosis. Subsequent urine organic acid analysis detected isovaleric acid and associated metabolites suggestive of isovaleric acidaemia.

In contrast to this typical neonatal onset acute metabolic presentation, IMD can also present with acute decompensation at a later stage, often precipitated by an intercurrent viral illness or other catabolic stress such as prolonged fasting, or surgical procedure.

IMD can also present with specific organ dysfunction, for example with cardiomyopathy, liver disease, seizure disorders, or developmental delay or regression. They are also a recognised cause of Sudden Unexplained Death in Infancy (SUDI).

The "storage disorders" do not cause acute metabolic crises, but are associated with a slowly progressive clinical phenotype often associated with dysmorphic features, organomegaly, skeletal dysplasia, or developmental regression. Specialised investigation of these disorders can include assessment of urine glycosaminoglycans, measurement of specific lysosomal enzyme activity in blood or skin cells, with second-line molecular genetic testing.

A number of important IMD are now detected through the Newborn Screening (NBS) programme. This aims to identify neonates at an early, pre-symptomatic stage and to facilitate the introduction of treatment to prevent acute illness. The universal NBS programme (Newborn Screening)in England now screens for six IMDs (Table 29.1). Heelprick blood spot card samples are collected on day five of life by the Midwife, and posted to the regional screening laboratory. Upon receipt the samples are processed, and any positive screening results are notified immediately to the appropriate metabolic team. This will then prompt contact to be made with the family, and depending on the condition, arrangements will either be made for immediate admission to the local paediatric unit for initial emergency management (for example for Maple syrup urine disease (MSUD)), or for review within a specified time frame in the metabolic clinic (for example for Phenylketonuria (PKU)). Further investigations are obtained to determine whether the initial screening result is a true positive. If the diagnosis is confirmed further management measures are continued, whereas if the diagnosis is not confirmed management will be normalised. All screening programmes aim to minimise "false positive" screening results. Occasionally, other medical conditions are picked up by blood spot test screening including beta-thalassaemia major, and some forms of tyrosinaemia and galactosaemia. However, the screening programme is not designed to reliably detect these conditions, and a normal NBS result does not exclude them.

NHS Newborn Bloodspot Screening Test
Sickle cell disease
Cystic fibrosis
Congenital hypothyroidism
Inherited metabolic disorders
Phenylketonuria (PKU)
Medium chain acylCoA dehydrogenase deficiency (MCADD)
Homocystinuria (Hcu)
Glutaric aciduria type 1 (GA-1)
Isovaleric acidaemia (IVA)
Maple syrup urine disease (MSUD)

Table 29.1: Conditions screened for as part of the UK newborn screening programme

Syllabus Mapping

Metabolism and Metabolic Medicine

- Know the common clinical presentations of metabolic disease

- Know about the screening procedures for inherited metabolic conditions

Neonatology

- Know about the range of newborn screening tests used in the UK including haematological and metabolic conditions, cystic fibrois and the universal newborn hearing screening programme

References and Further Reading

1. Clarke JTR, A clinical guide to Inherited Metabolic Diseases (3rd edition). Cambridge University Press 2006

2. www.bimdg.org.uk - British Inherited Metabolic Diseases Group : Emergency Guidelines for known and undiagnosed metabolic disorders. (Last accessed 14th July 2016)

Chapter 30: Choking when feeding
Dr Mithilesh Lal and Dr Nilesh Agrawal

Freya is a full term baby girl with a birth weight of 2588 grams who was discharged from the midwifery led maternity unit at 6 hours of age. She was thought to be well and stable at discharge. She was brought to the emergency department by her mother at 15 hours of age with breathing difficulties. Her mother says that she has been choking when she has tried to feed her on 4 occasions.

She was born at term by a normal delivery to a primiparous Caucasian mother who has type 1 diabetes. The 20 week anomaly scan showed normal fetal anatomy. During the pregnancy her mother drank 3-4 units of alcohol each week and measured "large for dates" on symphysis-fundal height. She presented with reduced fetal movements on 2 occasions at 36 weeks but had reassuring Cardiotocography (CTG) monitoring.

On examination Freya is pink and well perfused. Her temperature is 37.1^{0}C, heart rate 130/minute, respiratory rate 72/minute and oxygen saturations 97% in air. There is some frothing at the mouth and she has marked sub-costal and inter-costal recessions. Air entry is equal bilaterally with no added sounds. Her heart sounds are normal and her femoral pulses are easily palpable. There is no hepato-splenomegaly and she has good tone and a good suck. The nurse passes a nasogastric tube to 16 cm and obtains copious clear secretions.

Q1. What feature in this mother's pregnancy is most indicative of the underlying diagnosis?

A.   Drinking 3-4 units of alcohol each week
B.   Measuring "large for dates" on symphysis-fundal height measurement
C.   Normal fetal anomaly scan
D.   Reduced fetal movements at 36 weeks
E.   Type 1 diabetes mellitus

Q2. Which investigation is most likely to demonstrate the underlying diagnosis?

A.   Abdominal ultrasound scan
B.   Abdominal x-ray
C.   Chest x-ray
D.   Echocardiogram
E.   Test feed

Freya is listed for theatre.

Q3. What investigation is needed pre-operatively?

A.   Echocardiogram
B.   Limb x-ray
C.   Renal Ultrasound scan
D.   Serum cortisol
E.   Spinal ultrasound scan

Answers and Rationale

Q1.   B: Measuring "large for dates" on symphysis-fundal height measurement
Q2.   C: Chest x-ray
Q3.   A: Echocardiogram

Difficulty with feeding is common in the first few days of life. Often this is due to a combination of the babies in-coordinate feeding and mother's inexperience with a new baby. If the feeding doesn't appear to improve or there are features in the history suggestive of an underlying pathological disorder, as in Freyya's case, then the baby should be closely examined. This examination should focus on the following:

- Detection of a cleft palate (soft palate clefts can frequently be missed on the routine neonatal examination) by palpation and visual inspection of the entire palate with a light source and tongue depressor.
- Signs of respiratory distress, congenital heart disease or infection
- A dysmorphic syndrome (such as Down syndrome)
- Hypotonic disorder (e.g. Spinal Muscular Atrophy (SMA), Prader-Willi Syndrome). Neuromuscular conditions will present with hypotonia, and 'frog-leg' posture. Other associated features for example dysmorphism in Trisomy 21 or Prader Willi syndrome or tongue fasciculation's in SMA may provide pointers to the underlying diagnosis.
- Structural abnormalities such as oesophageal or choanal atresia. Unilateral choanal atresia can present with noisy breathing, feeding difficulty and choking. Bilateral choanal atresia will present at birth with cyanosis when not crying as babies are obligate nasal breathers. Passing an appropriate nasogastric tubes through both nostrils without difficulty will exclude this.

In Freya's case the clues to the underlying diagnosis are the antenatal history of mother measuring "large for dates", the frothing at the mouth and copious clear secretions from the nasogastric tube.

Measuring large for dates is indicative of a large baby or excessive amniotic fluid (polyhydramnios). This baby is small therefore making polyhydramnios the reason for measuring "large for dates". Causes of polyhdramnios are listed in table 30.1. The polyhydramnios along with having frothy secretions is commonly seen in oesphageal atresia.

Oesophageal atresia (OA) is a congenital abnormality in which there is a blind ending oesophagus. It can occur in isolation or there may be one or more fistulae communicating between the abnormal oesophagus and the trachea, known as a tracheo-oesophageal fistula (TOF) (1-3). In more than 50% of babies, oesophageal atresia is present with other anomalies. These include:

- VACTERL (Vertebral defects, Anorectal malformations, Cardiovascular defects, Tracheo-oesophageal defects, Renal abnormalities and Limb defects),
- CHARGE syndrome (Coloboma, Heart defects, Atresia choanae, Retarded development, Genital hypoplasia, Ear abnormalities),
- Trisomies 13, 18 and 21,
- Others: Pierre-Robin, Di George, Fanconi, and Polysplenia syndrome.

Antenatal presentation with maternal polyhydramnios and small or absent fetal stomach bubble on ultrasound scan has a sensitivity of 50%. Postnatally infants present in the first few hours of life with respiratory distress, choking, feeding difficulties and frothing at mouth. Passing of a nasogastric tube into the stomach is not possible because of the atresia however it may be passed into the blind ending oesophageal pouch where it curls up and can be seen on chest x-ray.

H-type fistula is where the osephagus is a continuum and connected to the stomach. They usually present later in infancy as there is no 'blind end' to the oesophagus and the child is able to feed, albeit with a recurrent cough or recurrent chest infections.

Initial management of oesophageal atresia is via surgical repair. Any fistula will be resected. If the two ends of the oesophagus can be brought together a primary repair is the preferred approach. If there is a long segment gap and the two ends cannot be brought together several approaches may be attempted. These include pulling the stomach into the chest, transposing the patients gut to bridge the gap or by inserting a gastrosomy to provide nutrition with an oesophagostomy to allow oesophageal secretions to drain and subsequently allowing the oesaphageal pouch to grow until re-anastamoses can be performed. Post-operative complications include anastamotic leak, stenosis at the ansatmotic site, oesophageal dysmotility and gastro-oesophageal reflux disease (GORD). A multidisciplinary approach involving surgeon, respiratory paediatrician, dietician, physiotherapist and speech therapist is appropriate to achieve good outcome.

Prior to surgery screening for associated abnormalities is important, particularly the detection of any congenital heart abnormalities which may require intervention prior and/during surgery. For example, a duct dependent heart lesion will require prostin to maintain ductal patency during surgery.

- Idiopathic (around 50% of all cases)

- Gastrointestinal anomalies impairing fetal swallowing - oesophageal atresia, duodenal atresia, congenital diaphragmatic hernia

- Fetal neuromuscular conditions e.g. SMA, myotonic dystrophy, anencephaly,

- Skeletal Dysplasia resulting in insufficient thoracic space to facilitate oesophageal development organ development

- Renal abnormalities resulting in fetal polyuria e.g. Bartter;'s syndrome

- Trisomy 21, 18, and 13

- Maternal diabetes

- Multiple pregnancy

- Fetal anaemia

- Congenital infections - toxoplasmosis, cytomegalovirus and rubella

- Hydrops fetalis

Table 30.1 Common causes of polyhydramnios (4-5)

Syllabus Mapping

Neonatology

- Know and understand the effects of antenatal and perinatal events

- Know the common minor congenital abnormalities and their initial management

- Know how to recognise, assess and initially manage respiratory disorders in the neonatal period

- Know about the identification, initial management and appropriate referral pathways for neonatal surgical problems including NEC

References

1. Pinheiro PF, Simoes e Silva AC, Pereira RM; Current knowledge on esophageal atresia. World J Gastroenterol. 2012 Jul 28; 18(28):3662-72. doi: 10.3748/wjg.v18.i28.3662

2. Goyal A, Jones MO, Couriel JM, Losty PD. Oesophageal atresia and tracheo-oesophageal fistula. Archives of Disease in Childhood-Fetal and Neonatal Edition. 2006 Sep 1;91(5):F381-4

3. Konkin DE, O'Hali WA, Webber EM, Blair GK. Outcomes in esophageal atresia and tracheoesophageal fistula. Journal of pediatric surgery. 2003 Dec 31;38(12):1726-9

4. Sandlin, Adam T., Suneet P. Chauhan, and Everett F. Magann. "Clinical relevance of sonographically estimated amniotic fluid volume polyhydramnios." Journal of Ultrasound in Medicine 32.5 (2013): 851-863

5. Hamza A, Herr D, Solomayer EF, Meyberg-Solomayer G. Polyhydramnios: causes, diagnosis and therapy. Geburtshilfe und Frauenheilkunde. 2013 Dec;73(12):1241-6

Further Reading

Parry RL. Selected gastrointestinal anomalies in the neonate. In: Martin RJ, Fanaroff AA, Walsh MC (Eds). Fanaroff and Martin's Neonatal-Perinatal Medicine: Diseases of the Fetus and Infant. 10th ed. Elsevier Saunders: 2015. P1395-1400

Sugarman I, Stringer MD, Smyth AG. Congenital defects and surgical problems. In Rennie JM (ed). Rennie and Robertson's Textbook of Neonatology. 5thed Churchill Livingstone Elsevier: 2012. P728-30

Chapter 31: Crash call to the emergency department
Dr Manjunath Ganga Shetty and Dr Poothirikovil Venugopalan

31

You are crash called urgently to the emergency department to attend to Rohan, a 7 day old baby boy who has been brought in via ambulance after he was found unresponsive 20 minutes ago by the parents. He was doing fine until last evening when his parents noted he was a bit off colour and did not take his feeds as well as usual. He was born at term weighing 3.5 kg and had a normal first day examination which included preductal and post ductal oxygen saturation screening. There were no risk factors for sepsis and he was discharged home at 8 hours of age.

On examination his airway is patent and he is receiving 100% oxygen via non-rebreathable mask. His respiratory rate is 20/minute with shallow respirations. His oxygen saturations are unreportable. His heart rate is 170/minute with capillary refill time of 4 seconds centrally. He is pale and mottled. His chest is clear and he has a 1/6 systolic murmur. The anaesthetist intubates and ventilates him. Venous blood gas results are: ph 6.99, BE -18 blood glucose of 3.4 mmol/l. You give him a 20 ml/kg bolus of saline and his heart rate is 150/minute with a capillary refill time of 2 seconds centrally.

Q1. What is the most important next management step?

A.   10 ml/kg bolus of saline
B.   20 ml/kg bolus of saline
C.   3 ml/kg of 10% dextrose
D.   Intravenous antibiotics
E.   Intravenous prostaglandin

Resuscitation continues and when he is stable a chest radiograph is performed showing an enlarged heart with pulmonary plethora. Despite 100% oxygen Rohan continues to have saturation of 70% and a repeat blood gas failed to show any significant improvement to the metabolic acidosis.

Q2. What is the most likely diagnosis?

A.   Congenital heart disease
B.   Diaphragmatic hernia
C.   Inherited metabolic disease
D.   Non-accidental Injury
E.   Sepsis

Q3. What would be the next most important management step?

A.   Intravenous bicarbonate
B.   Intravenous diuretics
C.   Intravenous ibuprofen
D.   Intravenous prostaglandin infusion
E.   Urgent echocardiogram

Answers and Rationale

Q1. **D: Intravenous antibiotics**
Q2. **A: Congenital heart disease**
Q3. **D: Intravenous prostaglandin infusion**

The commonest causes of collapse at this age are either due to sepsis, congenital heart disease or an inherited metabolic disorder. Systemic sepsis is the most common of these and is far more frequent than congenital cardiac conditions. Infants with accidental and non-accidental injuries can also present similarly and this needs to be considered. A good history and clinical examination with high index of suspicion help in the prompt diagnosis and effective management of babies presenting in this way. The initial resuscitation of a baby presenting in a collapsed state should be as per the basic life support and advanced paediatric life support. Once stabilised, given that sepsis is the most likely cause of sudden post-natal collapse it is critical that the urgent administration of antibiotics occurs. In this case, the most likely initial diagnosis is sepsis. A soft systolic murmur is not uncommon in the first few days of life and does not indicate a congenital heart defect is present. Most murmurs are either innocent flow murmurs or related to the closure of the arterial duct and/or foramen ovale.

Despite high oxygen administration and adequate ventilation, Rohan's perfusion and oxygenation does not improve. A significant metabolic acidosis persists and the chest radiograph is indicative of an underlying cardiac defect with enlarged cardiac silhouette and pulmonary plethora. Given this additional information the most likely cause for Rohan's collapse is actually congenital heart disease. This is a situation that is relatively common and highlights the need to re-visit a diagnosis if the clinical picture doesn't fit with your original thoughts. A normal newborn examination does not exclude a significant congenital heart disease as transition from fetal to neonatal circulation makes clinical assessment of the heart less reliable. Furthermore, clinical recognition of cyanosis is difficult in newborn babies and heart murmurs may be soft or absent even in the presence of a critical heart disease. Femoral pulses may be palpable as the arterial duct may remain patent. Nevertheless, it is important to listen to Rohan's heart sounds and for the presence of murmurs, and to palpate peripheral pulses including femoral pulses for volume and character. His blood pressure should be monitored. Where abnormal, these could give a clue to an underlying heart disease.

More recently, routine oxygen saturation monitoring has formed part of the routine newborn screening examination. Pulse oximetry measurements in the right arm (preductal) and right/left leg (postductal) help to identify heart disease in the newborn. Preliminary results are encouraging, although this technique is not without fallacy either. The method is more reliable in the presence of right heart obstructive diseases (pulmonary atresia) compared to the left heart obstructive diseases (coarctation of the aorta) (1). Once the diagnosis of a congenital heart defect is considered we need to urgently initiate therapy to restore blood flow to the lungs and/or body. Congenital heart defects presenting at this age usually do so as the arterial duct, which has been supporting systemic or pulmonary blood flow, is closing. Prostaglandin infusion has to be started immediately to maintain patency or to open up the arterial duct. Facilities for an immediate echocardiogram may not be available in many centres and there should not be delay in starting prostaglandin infusion whilst waiting for a cardiology opinion or echocardiogram, even when in-house echocardiogram facilities are available.Prostaglandin infusion would prevent the arterial duct from closing and would re-establish patency if closure has already occurred and thereby increase PaO_2, and mitigate metabolic acidosis. This drug is indicated as a temporary management for the neonate with duct dependant congenital heart disease while awaiting transfer to a cardiac centre. Duct dependant congenital heart diseases are discussed below.

Critical congenital heart diseases (CHD) in the newborn:

Critical CHD presenting within the first few weeks of life constitute 15% of CHD and have a high associated mortality and morbidity (2). Antenatal screening by ultrasound and postnatal screening using preductal and postductal oxygen saturations help in recognising some of these conditions even when they are asymptomatic as explained above. These life threatening heart conditions may not have obvious evidence early after birth and most of the clinical and physical findings are nonspecific in these babies. Sepsis, persistent pulmonary hypertension of newborn, respiratory and metabolic conditions can present similarly. A high index of suspicion and astute acumen are essential in managing these critically unwell babies.

Pathophysiology:

Before birth the fetal circulation differs from ex-utero life as the placenta is the organ for oxygenation and not the lungs. The fetal lungs therefore only receive a small volume of blood with the need for the rest of the de-oxygenated blood in the right ventricle to return to the placenta. This is achieved by the arterial duct allowing the blood to flow from the pulmonary artery to the descending aorta. Where there is an obstruction to the left ventricular outflow (coarctation of the aorta, hypoplastic left heart) or to the right ventricular outflow (pulmonary atresia), or where the great arteries are connected to the wrong ventricles (transposition of the great arteries), the presence of the arterial duct and foramen ovale ensure that the pulmonary and systemic circulations are maintained and effective in the delivery of oxygenated blood to the body. These critical heart diseases therefore do not generally manifest symptoms in utero and the same situation continues for a few days after birth. With the natural closure of the arterial duct in the first week of life, there is a sudden change to this arrangement, and the baby can deteriorate and collapse within a few hours of birth, generally between days 3 to day 7 of life. Prompt recognition of the underlying cardiac defect and re-opening the arterial duct with prostaglandin infusion is lifesaving.

Left-sided obstructive lesions:

In neonates with severe left-sided obstructive lesions the systemic blood flow is entirely or partly dependent on right-to-left flow through patent arterial duct. Conditions include coarctation of aorta (CoA), hypoplastic left heart syndrome (HLHS), critical aortic stenosis and interrupted aortic arch.

Coarctation of the Aorta:

Coarctation of the Aorta constitutes 8 to 10% of all CHD, and is characterised by a narrowing of the descending thoracic aorta adjacent to the point where the ductus arteriosus joins. As part of cardiovascular examination it is important to feel the femoral pulses as in this condition they may be weak or absent, though right upper limb pulses are normally palpable. Pulse oximetry may be helpful in the early diagnosis. Definitive treatment is surgical resection of the narrow segment and end-to-end anastomosis to relieve the obstruction.

Hypoplastic Left Heart Syndrome (HLHS):
HLHS is rare and accounts for 9% of the critically ill infants with congenital heart disease. HLHS includes a group of closely related anomalies characterized by hypoplasia of the left ventricle, atresia or critical stenosis of aortic valve and/or mitral valve and hypoplasia of the ascending aorta and aortic arch. CoA is frequently an associated finding. The only way blood can enter aorta and rest of the body is through the arterial duct. Univentricular circulation, where one ventricle would support both pulmonary and systemic circulations can be achieved in a staged surgical approach.

Right-sided obstructive lesions:
In neonates with severe right sided obstructive lesions, pulmonary blood flow is dependent on patency of the arterial duct. Conditions include pulmonary atresia and tricuspid atresia.

Pulmonary atresia:
Pulmonary atresia is rare and accounts for 2.5% of the critically ill infants with congenital heart disease. Pulmonary circulation is dependent on arterial duct flow from left to right. Severe cyanosis and tachyopnea are present from early life. Besides a prostaglandin infusion to keep the duct open, surgery to create a systemic to pulmonary shunt (Blalock-Taussig shunt) may be required.

Tricuspid atresia:
Constitutes 1 to 3% of congenital heart disease. The tricuspid valve is absent with absence of the inflow to the hypoplastic right ventricle. Associated defects like ASD, VSD and or PDA is essential for survival. Cyanosis is present from birth. Besides opening up the ductus arteriosus, balloon atrial septostomy could be considered to augment the atrial communication and staged surgical procedures to achieve a univentricular circulation planned.

Transposition of great arteries (TGA):
Here, the aorta arises from right ventricle and pulmonary artery from left ventricle. Arterial duct and foramen ovale patency help to ensure adequate mixing of systemic and pulmonary blood flows. Besides keeping the ductus arteriosus open, almost all babies require balloon atrial septostomy to ensure adequate mixing of blood. Surgical switch of the aorta and pulmonary artery with transplantation of the coronary arteries form the corrective surgery.

Syllabus Mapping

Cardiology

- Know the clinical features of common congenital heart conditions and understand the principle of management

- Know the value of oxygen saturation measurement in the assessment of possible congenital heart disease

Neonatology

- Be able to recognise and initiate the management of common disorders in the newborn including sepsis

- Know the range of newborn screening tests used in the UK including haematological and metabolic conditions, cystic fibrosis and the universal newborn hearing screening programme

Emergency Medicine (including accidents and poisoning)

- Be able to recognise and provide initial management for life threatening airway, breathing or circulatory compromise

Infection, Immunology and Allergy

- Know when antimicrobials are indicated

References

1. Ismail AQ, Cawsey M, Ewer AK. Newborn pulse oximetry screening in practice. Archives of Disease in Childhood-Education & Practice edition. 2016 Aug 16:edpract-2016

2. Wren, Christopher, Zdenka Reinhardt, and Khuloud Khawaja. "Twenty-year trends in diagnosis of life-threatening neonatal cardiovascular malformations". Archives of Disease in Childhood-Fetal and Neonatal Edition 93.1 (2008): F33-F35

Further Reading

Park MK, Park's Pediatric Cardiology for Practitioners, 6th Edition, 2014, Elsevier Saunders Publication

Chapter 32: Advice to a new mum
Dr Satyam Veeratterapillay
and Dr Mithilesh Lal

(32)

You perform a routine baby check on a term baby boy at 24 hours of age. He was born by a normal vaginal delivery at term, to a primiparous mother with no risk factors for infection. This was an uneventful pregnancy and his mother has no medical history but she smokes 10 cigarettes each day. She states that her baby is not breast feeding well and has had several possets. Her friend's child who was born at 32 weeks died of "cot death" at 4 months of age and he was formula fed. She is worried about her baby and wants advice about reducing the risk of "cot death".

Q1. At what age is the greatest risk of SIDS (sudden infant death syndrome)?

A.   0-14 days
B.   14-28 days
C.   2-4 months
D.   4-6 months
E.   6-12 months

Q2. The mother wants advice about feeding. She asks what effect switching to formula milk will have on the risk of "cot death".

A.   No effect
B.   There is a significant decreased risk
C.   There is a significant increased risk
D.   There is a small decreased risk
E.   There is a small increased risk

The mother asks you what she should do regarding his sleeping position if he continues to posset milk at home.

Q3. What is your advice?

A.   Put him to sleep on his back
B.   Put him to sleep on his side
C.   Put him to sleep prone
D.   Swaddle him
E.   Use an apnoea alarm

She asks if preterm babies are more likely to die from "cot death".

Q4. Which one of these options best describes the risk of SIDS in preterm infants as compared to infants born at term?

A.   2 times increase in risk
B.   4 times increase in risk
C.   8 times increase in risk
D.   10 times increase in risk
E.   No increase in risk

Answers and Rationale

Q1. **C: 2-4 months**
Q2. **C: There is a significant increased risk**
Q3. **A: Put him to sleep on his back**
Q4. **B: 4 times increase in risk**

Sudden infant death syndrome (SIDS) refers to the sudden, unexpected death of an infant less than 1 year of age, with the onset of the lethal episode apparently occurring during sleep, which remains unexplained after a thorough investigation, including a complete post-mortem examination and review of the circumstances of death (1). Although the incidence has reduced significantly over the recent decades, SIDS remains the leading cause of infant death in Western countries, contributing to almost 50% of post neonatal deaths (1). As such, it remains a source of great anxiety for parents and it is important for health professionals to give accurate advice on the proposed mechanism, risk factors and protective strategies to mitigate such risks.

Mechanism

The triple risk hypothesis (fig 32.1) proposes that SIDS may occur when a vulnerable infant, such as one born preterm or exposed to maternal smoking, is at a critical but unstable developmental period in homeostatic control and is exposed to an exogenous stressor, such as being placed prone to sleep (2). SIDS usually occurs during sleep, with a peak in incidence between 2 and 4 months of age, when sleep patterns are rapidly maturing. The final pathway to SIDS is widely believed to involve immature cardiorespiratory control in conjunction with a failure of arousal from sleep (3).

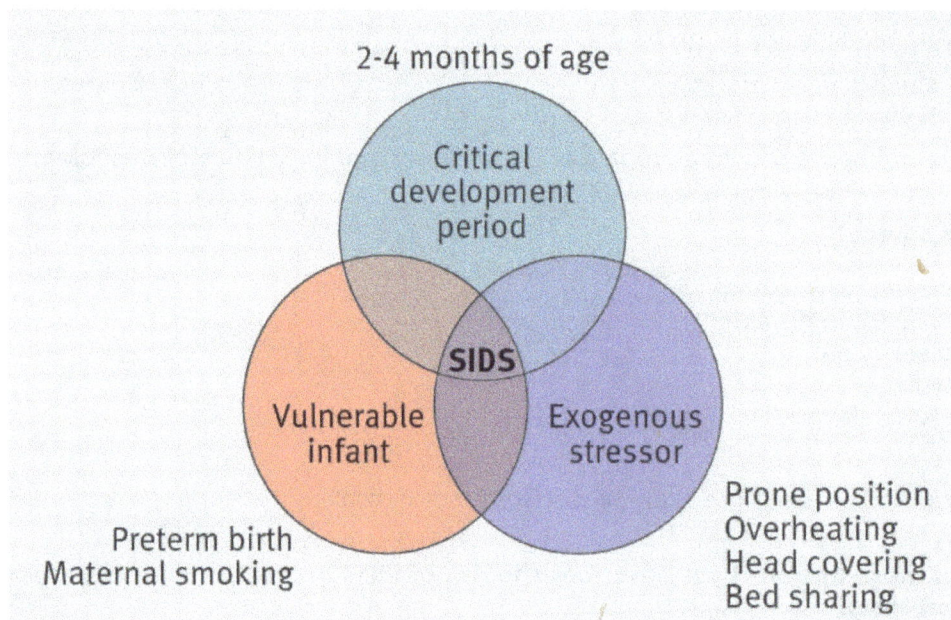

Figure 32.1: Triple risk model for sudden infant death syndrome (SIDS) illustrating three overlapping factors: vulnerable infant, critical developmental period and exogenous stressors. (Adapted from 2)

Pathology

There are no pathognomonic autopsy findings, although petechial haemorrhages, pulmonary oedema and structural evidence of chronic, low grade asphyxia are commonly seen (4). Brainstem abnormalities include abnormalities within medullary respiratory centres, and 5-hydroxytryptamine (5-HT or serotonin) receptors of the arcuate nucleus. Serotonin is an important neurotransmitter and is involved in influencing respiratory drive and arousal, cardiovascular control, thermoregulation, and upper airway reflexes. Altered serotonin homeostasis may therefore create an underlying vulnerability contributing to SIDS (4).

Risk factors, protective factors and advice: Risk factors from multiple studies on infants with SIDS include:

1. **Pregnancy-related risk factors:** Multiple gestation, prematurity, low birth weight and intrauterine growth restriction all are associated with higher incidence of SIDS (4). Preterm infants have a fourfold increased risk as compared to their term counterparts, and parents should be counselled about this prior to discharge (1).

2. **Cigarette smoking:** Intrauterine exposure to cigarette smoke increases the risk of SIDS up to fivefold. Studies have also shown that the risk of SIDS increases with daily cigarette use and exposure to environmental tobacco smoke (5). As a result, parents should be encouraged to reduce smoking as much as possible during pregnancy and after birth and to discourage smoking around the baby.

3. **Drug and alcohol use:** Prenatal drug use, especially opiates, has been linked with increased risk of SIDS. While prenatal and post-natal alcohol use has not been associated with SIDS, some studies have also found that maternal consumption of alcohol in the 24 hours prior the infant's death carried a 2 to 8-fold increased risk of SIDS (4). Parents should be encouraged to avoid the use of alcohol and illicit drugs.

4. **Sleeping position:** Prone sleeping position has been consistently shown to increase the risk of SIDS (1). Side sleeping was also identified as a risk factor, likely due to the relative instability of this position and infants rolling to a prone position during sleep. The current recommendation is for supine position for sleeping ("back to sleep") for all infants except those few with specific medical conditions for which recommending a different position may be justified (6). It is important to reassure parents who are concerned about the risk of choking in supine position, as evidence shows that the risk of regurgitation and choking is highest in prone-sleeping infants.

5. **Sleeping place:** Sleeping on a sofa or couch increases the risk of SIDS 67-fold. (1) Parents should be counselled about this and advised that it is riskier to feed their baby on a sofa than on a bed. Moreover, bed sharing- a situation where an adult (typically one or both parents) brings the infant on to the same surface (usually, but not limited to, a mattress) for sleep has been associated with an increased risk of SIDS. (1) While it is a common practice in many healthcare settings, the current recommendations are that infants aged less than 6 months should sleep in their own cot and not share a sleeping surface with a parent, caregiver, or other child (6).

6. **Bed surfaces and bedding:** Soft bedding increases the risk of SIDS, and infants with SIDS were more likely to have been found with their head covered by loose bedding. (1) Infants should be placed to sleep on a firm, well-fitting mattress which is flat. Parents should avoid using any loose or soft bedding that could cover an infant's face such as heavy blankets, pillows, or cot bumpers, and should not place toys in the cot. If blankets are used, infants should be placed with their feet at the foot of the cot and the blanket tucked in on three sides to reduce the risk of the head becoming covered. A good alternative to blankets is an infant sleeping bag (6).

7. **Temperature:** Studies have shown that overheating was associated with increased risk of SIDS. This may be related to a failure of thermal autoregulation or the fact that babies in the prone position tend to have a higher body temperature. Parents are advised to keep their baby not too warm, nor too cold and to avoid placing the cot next to a radiator or heat source, and making sure their heads are not covered by bedclothes or hats when they are asleep indoors (4).

The following factors which have been shown to protect against the risk of SIDS:

1. **Breast feeding:** breast feeding has been linked with reduced risk reduction of SIDS by 50% (1). The protective effective was strongest with exclusive breast feeding. Parents should therefore be strongly encouraged to breastfeed for this as well as other health benefits (4).
2. **Room sharing:** Infants sleeping in their own cot in the parental bedroom were found to have reduced risk of SIDS by 50%. This is likely due to parents being able to closely monitor their children and therefore reduce the risk of suffocation, strangulation or entrapment (1). Parents should be advised to room share for the first 6 to 12 months (4).
3. **Pacifiers:** There is strong evidence that children dying from SIDS were less likely to have used a pacifier during their last sleep. While some countries advocate the use of pacifiers as a risk reduction strategy for SIDS, this is not the case in the UK. Parents wanting to breastfeed should avoid its use in the first 3-4 weeks when breastfeeding is being established (1).

Advice to expectant parents following SIDS related death
The next born siblings of infants dying of any non-infectious natural cause are at significantly increased risk for infant death from the same cause, including SIDS. There is a 9 fold increased risk for the same cause of death. This increased risk in families who have experienced SIDS is consistent with genetic factors interacting with environmental risk factors (4).Parents enquiring about home monitoring equipment (apnoea alarm, respiratory, cardiac, oxygen saturation monitoring) should be advised that numerous studies have shown that there is no decreased risk of SIDS in infants using these (4). Home monitoring equipment is therefore not recommended to prevent SIDS, although it may be appropriate in select group of infants (e.g. complex patients on long term ventilation) (6).

Having an infant death from SIDS is an extremely traumatic experience for any parent. In the UK, the care of next infant (CONI) programme aims to support these parents by offering regular health check reviews, emphasising safe sleeping practices, feeding advice and avoiding prenatal and postnatal exposure to tobacco smoke.

Syllabus Mapping

Respiratory

* Know the role of health promotion programmes in preventing sudden infant death and be able to advise parents on avoiding risks

Nutrition

* Understand the principles of infant feeding

References

1. Horne RSC, Hauch FR. Sudden infant death syndrome and advice for safe sleeping. BMJ 2015; 350:h1989

2. Filiano JJ, Kinney HC. A perspective on neuropathologic findings in victims of the sudden infant death syndrome: the triple-risk model. Neonatology. 1994 Jul 1;65(3-4):194-7

3. Moon RY, Home RS, Hauch FR. Sudden infant death syndrome. Lancet 2007; 370:1578-87

4. Hunt CE, Hauck FR. Sudden Infant Death Syndrome. In: Kliegman RM, Stanton BF (eds) Nelson Textbook of Pediatrics 19th edition. Elsevier Saunders 2011: 1424-25

5. Dwyer T, Ponsonby AL, Couper D. Tobacco smoke exposure at one month of age and subsequent risk of SIDS—a prospective study. American Journal of Epidemiology. 1999 Apr 1;149(7):593-602

6. American Academy of Pediatrics Task force on Sudden Infant Death Syndrome. SIDS and other sleep-related infant deaths: expansion of recommendations for a safe infant sleeping environment. Pediatrics 2011; 128; e1341

Further reading

Martin RJ, Fanaroff AA. Fanaroff and Martin's neonatal-perinatal medicine: diseases of the fetus and infant 9th edition. Elsevier Saunders 2011: 1145-46

Rennie JM. Rennie and Robertsons' textbook of neonatology 5th edition. Churchill Livingstone 2012:578

Chapter 33: The changing ECG
Dr Poothirikovil Venugopalan and Dr Manjunath Ganga Shetty

33

You are seeing patients in the children's outpatient clinic. Your next patient is a 14 year old girl, Claire, who attends with the following referral letter from her GP:

"This young lady presents with a 2-month history of intermittent palpitations. These have been occurring at rest and last for 5-10 minutes. There is no history of chest pain, dizziness or syncope. She had an episode of palpitation while in the Surgery and I have managed to record an ECG during the episode (please see attached – Figure 33.1). Her family is concerned as one of her cousins died of a heart defect in the first week of life."

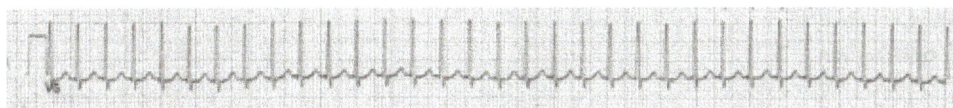

Figure 33.1: ECG rhythm strip recorded by the GP

On examination she is pink, well perfused, with normal growth and development. There is no clinical evidence of thyroid dysfunction. She has normal peripheral pulses, her blood pressure 120/80 mmHg, normal heart sounds and no heart murmur. Her chest is clear to auscultation, and abdomen is soft with no organomegaly. You perform an ECG in clinic. (Figure 33.2).

Figure 33.2: ECG rhythm strip performed in clinic at same scale as ECG in 33.1

Here is a list of diagnoses, choose the most appropriate answer for each question:

A.	Atrial tachycardia	F.	Supraventricular tachycardia
B.	Prolonged QT syndrome	G.	Ventricular ectopics
C.	Sinus arrhythmia	H.	Ventricular fibrillation
D.	Sinus bradycardia	I.	Ventricular tachycardia
E.	Sinus tachycardia	J.	Wolff Parkinson White Syndrome

Q1a. What does the ECG taken in the GP Surgery (Figure 33.1) show?

Q1b. What does the ECG taken in the clinic (Figure 33.2) show?

Q1c. What is the most likely cause of Claire's palpitations?

Answers and Rationale

Q1a. **F: Supraventricular tachycardia**
Q1b. **C: Sinus arrhythmia**
Q1c. **F: Supraventricular tachycardia**

To answer this question, we should revisit the basics of interpreting a paediatric ECG. A systematic approach includes assessing the rhythm (Is this sinus rhythm?), rate, axis of P wave and QRS complex, individual components (P wave, QRS complex and T wave) and intervals (PR, QRS, QTc). (Figure 33.3) gives an overview of the different waves and measurements.

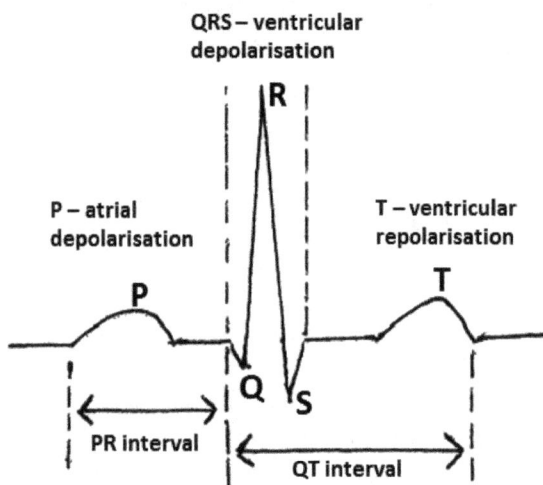

Figure: 33.3. ECG waves and measurements

Sinus rhythm is when all the cardiac cycles are triggered from sinus node and this is evident on the ECG when each QRS complex is preceded by a P wave, and the P wave is upright in lead 1 and aVF. The QRS axis represents the mean electrical axis of ventricular depolarisation and is calculated using any 2 limb leads. The PR, QRS and QT intervals should be measured. The QT interval varies with heart rate and Bazett's formula (QT/$\sqrt{RR}$) is used to calculate the corrected QT interval for a given heart rate (1).

In this scenario the ECG recorded by the GP (Figure 33.1) shows no P waves, with a regular, but extremely rapid heart rate of more than 200/minute. The QRS complexes are of normal duration and configuration. These findings are suggestive of supraventricular tachycardia (SVT). The ECG recorded in clinic (Figure 33.2) shows P waves preceding all QRS complexes. The P wave is upright indicating sinus rhythm. There is a gradual variation in the RR interval (i.e. heart rate) with maintenance of the sinus rhythm characteristic. The rate is 72/minute (300 divided by the number of large squares between two R waves). The PR interval (from the beginning of the P wave to the beginning of the QRS complex) is 130 milliseconds, QRS duration (beginning of the Q wave to the end of the S wave) is 50 milliseconds and the QTc is 410 msec. This ECG is consistent with sinus arrhythmia. Sinus arrhythmia is a normal phasic variation in the heart rate, increasing during inspiration and decreasing during expiration. This is due to the variation in the activity of the autonomic nerves with the different phases of respiration. This girl is therefore having paroxysmal attacks of

SVT which are the cause of her palpitations. It must be noted however that palpitations in children are more often non-cardiac in origin (see Table 33.1). A careful history and examination may suggest the cause of the palpitations though often a 24 hour tape or an event recorder is required to document the arrhythmia.

Physiological	Exercise, Excitement, Fever
Psychogenic	Stress, Anxiety disorders, Panic attacks
Cardiac	Arrhythmias Congenital heart disease Postsurgical Cardiomyopathies Cardiac tumours or Infiltrative conditions
Other medical conditions	Anaemia, Throtoxicosis, Hypoglycaemia
Drugs	Caffeine, Smoking, Catecholamines, Theophylline, Beta-blockers, Antihypertensives, Antiarrythmic drugs, Cocaine

Table 33.1: Causes of palpitation in children

SVT is the most common abnormal cardiac rhythm disturbance in children, which requires treatment. The characteristics on ECG include a regular rhythm, fast heart rate (>210/minute in infants and >180/minute beyond infancy), narrow QRS complex and absence of p waves (or abnormal p waves when identifiable). The history is important to exclude any other causes of tachycardia, such as fever or dehydration etc, especially when the heart rate is near the upper end of the normal. SVT is generally well tolerated. If the SVT is persistent, or causes haemodynamic disturbance, emergency management aims to achieve sinus rhythm by slowing atrioventricular conduction. An intravenous bolus of adenosine is the recommended treatment. While procuring adenosine, vagal manoeuvres (ice cold water on the face, carotid sinus massage, Valsalva manoeuvre etc) can sometimes revert the SVT to sinus rhythm without the need for a medication (2). The underlying mechanism in SVT in most children is the presence of an accessory pathway that can transmit the cardiac impulse between the atria and the ventricles. In a majority of children with SVT, this accessory pathway is inactive, and starts conducting only at the time when the child goes into SVT. In a small number of the children with SVT, the pathway is however active during sinus rhythm, and can be identified on a 12 lead ECG by the presence of a short PR interval, delta wave and apparent prolongation of the QRS complex (secondary to the early take off of the delta wave) (Figure 33.4). The ECG pattern when the accessory pathway can be demonstrated on a 12 lead ECG is referred to as Wolf Parkinson White syndrome (3).

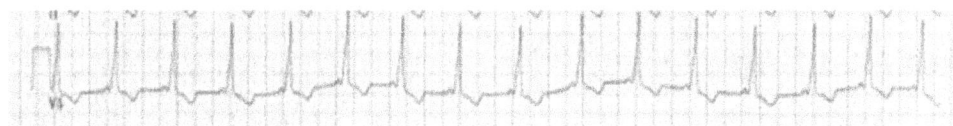

Figure 33.4: ECG showing a short PR interval (40 milliseconds), presence of a delta waves (initial slurring of QRS complex), and an apparent prolongation of the QRS complex (120 milliseconds) – features consistent with Wolf Parkinson White syndrome

Prevention of SVT depends on the age of the child and frequency of symptoms. A 'no treatment' approach can be accepted with infrequent self-terminating episodes in older children. Beta adrenergic blockers are effective in prevention, and are especially used in neonates and infants who cannot verbalise their symptoms and who have less cardiac reserve compared to older children. Radiofrequency ablation of the accessory pathway after mapping the pathway by electrophysiological studies is the treatment of choice in older children with frequent episodes of SVT (3).The important differential diagnosis for SVT is sinus tachycardia (ST), which refers to a heart rate that is above the normal upper limit for the age of the child. With ST the ECG waves retain the features of a sinus rhythm. Causes include anxiety, fever, anaemia, hypovolaemia/circulatory shock and thyrotoxicosis. It is worth remembering that heart failure can also cause sinus tachycardia, so just the identification of sinus tachycardia on an ECG does not rule out heart disease.A less common, but more serious cardiac arrhythmia in children is ventricular tachycardia (VT), identified on an ECG by the broad QRS complexes, absence of a regular p wave before the QRS complex and a bizarre pattern of the QRS complex with the R wave and S wave being in opposite directions (Figure 33.5). Where a p wave can be identified it bears no relationship to the QRS complex (atrio-ventricular dissociation), a hallmark of ventricular tachycardia.

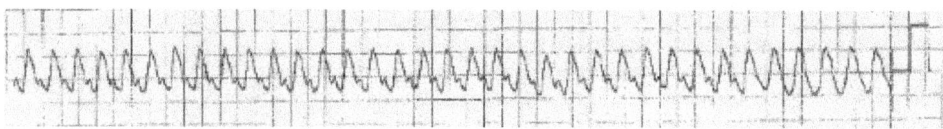

Figure 33.5: ECG showing ventricular tachycardia

Syllabus mapping

Cardiology

- Know the clinical features of common congenital heart conditions and understand the priniciples of management

- Know the common causes of palpitations and syncope and chest pain, know when to refer

Emergency Medicine (including accidents and poisoning)

- Be able to recognise and provide initial management for life threatening airway, breathing or circulatory collapse

References and Further Reading

1. Park MK, Guntheroth WG. How to read pediatric ECGs, 4th Edition, 2006, Mosby Elsevier Publication, Philadelphia, USA

2. Samuels M, Wieteska M. Advanced Paediatric Life Support, The Practical Approach, Fifth Edition, 2012, Wiley-Blackwell Publication, Chichester, UK

3. Park MK, Park's Pediatric Cardiology for Practitioners, 6th Edition, 2014, Elsevier Saunders Publication, Philadelphia, USA

Chapter 34: "Her snoring keeps the family awake!"
Dr Priya Kumar and Dr Chris Dewhurst

34

You see Risha, a 12 year old girl of Asian origin with her parents in clinic. Her GP has referred her to clinic as her asthma symptoms have not been well controlled on occasional use of a salbutamol inhaler and twice daily use of a steroid inhaler. She is tired during the day and has missed a total of 3 weeks of school in the past 3 months. She has mild learning difficulties. Her mother reports that she snores loudly at night and has had several episodes of otitis media. Her mother has type 2 diabetes mellitus and her father has hypertension.

On examination her height and weight are both greater than the 99.6th centile. Her respiratory rate is 30/ minute and she has a wheeze heard bilaterally. She has violaceous striae on her thighs and abdomen, lines of hyper pigmented, thickened skin on the back of her neck and has moderate acne on her face.

Her mother is concerned that her weight is impacting on her current health.

Q1. Which of the following health problem(s) is linked to Risha's obesity?

A.   Acne and being tired during the day
B.   Acne and otitis media
C.   Asthma and acne
D.   Asthma, acne and being tired during the day
E.   Asthma, acne, being tired during the day and otitis media

Q2. Which of the following factors is unlikely to be a risk factor for the development of obesity?

A.   Asian Ethnicity
B.   Learning difficulties
C.   Mother with Type 2 Diabetes Mellitus
D.   Prolonged use of a steroid inhaler
E.   Small for gestational age

Q3. Which of the following is the most likely going to have a positive impact impact upon Risha's obesity?

A.   Having semi-skimmed milk
B.   Referring Risha and her parents to a weight management programme
C.   Referring Risha to a weight management programme
D.   Stopping the steroid inhaler
E.   Watching TV for a maximum of 1 hour per day

Answers and Rationale

Q1.   D: Asthma, acne and being tired during the day
Q2.   D: Prolonged use of a steroid inhaler
Q3.   B: Referring Risha and her parents to a weight management programme

The World Health Organization (WHO) regards childhood obesity as one of the most serious global public health challenges for the 21st century. Recent data has shown that 1 in 3 children aged 10-11 in the UK are obese or overweight (1). In addition, younger generations are becoming obese at earlier ages and staying obese for longer (2). Obese children and adolescents are at an increased risk of developing various health problems, and are also more likely to become obese adults. It is estimated that reducing obesity levels will save lives as being obese doubles the risk of dying prematurely (3). The economic costs of obesity are also great. It was estimated that the NHS in England spent £5.1 billion on overweight and obesity-related ill-health in 2014/15 (4). Obesity is therefore a huge public health issue and in 2016 the UK government produced a plan for action on childhood obesity. This included legislative changes to tax on sugary drinks, reduce the sugar content of foods by 20%, promoting healthy eating and increasing children's activity and involvement with sports (5).

When faced with a child who appears to be overweight you must first take accurate measurements of weight and height and determine their body mass index. Assessing the body mass index (BMI) of children is more complicated than for adults because it changes as they grow and mature. Thresholds that take into account a child's age and sex are used to assess whether their BMI is too high or too low. These are usually derived from a reference population with the data presented in BMI centile charts. In a clinical assessment, a child on or above the 98th centile is classified as obese and between the 91st and 98th centile is classified as overweight (6). Other anthropometric measurements include skin fold thickness, waist circumference, waist to hip ratio and bio-impedance.

Obesity most commonly will not have an underlying medical cause and is known as "simple obesity" (Box 34.1). Rarely there will be an underlying medical diagnosis causing obesity. (Table 34.2) from (6)).

Simple obesity is a complex problem with many drivers, including behaviour, environment, genetics and culture. However, at its root obesity is caused by an energy imbalance: taking in more energy through food than we use through activity. Factors associated with the development of simple obesity are included in box 34.1.

- lack of education about food
- limited cooking skills
- limited money to buy healthier food to
- longer working hours
- marketing campaigns for junk food aimed at kids.
- sedentary lives children lead
- TV/ computer games
- 'clean your plate' syndrome (portion size)

Box 34.1: Factors associated with development of "Simple Obesity" (6)

Obese children are more likely to be ill, be absent from school due to illness, experience health-related limitations and require more medical care than normal weight children. Overweight and obese children are also more likely to become obese adults, and have a higher risk of morbidity, disability and premature mortality in adulthood (5). The children suffer from low self-esteem, bullying, depression and obesity related illness such as Type 2 Diabetes and obstructive sleep apnoea which is present in Risha manifested by her being tired during the day and snoring excessively. There is conflicting evidence about the prevalence of acne in obesity however the largest study has confirmed that there is an association in girls but not in boys (7). A recent meta-analysis concluded that overweight and obese children are at a 40-50% increased risk of asthma compared to normal weight children (8) with other studies suggesting that a higher BMI to contributes more severe asthma (9).

Condition	Differentiating signs/symptoms		Differentiating investigations
Primary Hypothyroidism	• Fatigue • Attenuated growth • Cold intolerance • Constipation	• Declining school performance • Dry skin • Coarse hair • Goitre	• Low free T4 low for age • Thyrotropin (TSH) will be elevated for age
Secondary hypothyroidism	• Fatigue • Poor growth • Cold intolerance	• Constipation • Dry skin • Coarse hair	• Free T4 low for age • TSH low or normal
Cushing's syndrome	• Attenuated growth • Violaceous striae • Buffalo hump • Central adiposity	• Moon facies • Hirsutism • Hypertension • Diabetes	• Elevated 24-hour urinary free cortisol is elevated
Prader-Willi syndrome	• Short stature • Small hands and feet • Almond-shaped eyes • Picking on skin	• Delayed puberty • Developmental delay • Hyperphagia • Poor feeding and hypotonia as infant	• Genetic testing shows imprinting error on chromosome 15
Bardet-Biedl syndrome	• Dysmorphic extremities • Retinitis pigmentosa	• Developmental delay • Hypogonadism • Renal defects	• Genetic testing

Condition	Differentiating signs/ symptoms	Differentiating investigations	Condition
Pseudohypo-parathyroidism	• Short stature • Round face • Short metacarpals	• Developmental delay • Basal ganglia calcification	• Hypocalcaemia • hyperphosphataemia • Elevated PTH
Monogenic obesity	• Severe, early-onset obesit	• Disruption of normal appetite control mechanisms	• Mutations in MC4-R gene most common
Hypothalamic obesity	• following treatment for intracranial lesions	• Excessive appetite	• Abnormal hypo -thalamopituitary testing
Obesity due to medication	• Neuropsychiatric drugs • Corticosteroids	• Others	• Discontinuation of drug as a therapeutic trial

Table 34.2 Medical causes of obesity (6)

Recent guidance has advocated the use of lifestyle weight management programmes which focus on diet, physical activity and behaviour-change. Some programmes will aim to maintain the growing child's existing weight in the short term, as they grow taller often described as 'growing into their weight'. Young people who are overweight or obese and are no longer growing taller will ultimately need to lose weight to improve their BMI. These changes then need to become firmly established habits over the long term. Involving the wider family in these programmes is more likely to be successful than just involving the child (10).

Syllabus Mapping

Endocrinology and Growth

- Know the presentation of disorders of the adrenal, thyroid and parathyroid glands and understand the principles of management

- Know the presentation of disorders of the pituitary gland and understand the principles of management

- Understand the principles and practice of growth measurement, including plotting and interpretation of growth charts

- Know the causes of abnormal growth including short stature and slow or accelerated growth. Know about appropriate assessment, investigation and treatment

Nutrition

- Know the causes of malnutrition and understand the epidemiology and public health consequences of obesity

- Be able to recognise obesity, understand the consequences of obesity on health and well-being in the short and long term and advise young people and their families on effective strategies to manage this and use BMI measurements and charts

References and Further Reading

1. Statistics on Obesity, Physical Activity and Diet. England, 2016. United Kingdom Statistics Authority published April 28th 2016

2. Johnson W, Li L, Kuh D, Hardy R (2015) How Has the Age-Related Process of Overweight or Obesity Development Changed over Time?. PLoS Med 12(5)

3. T. Pischon, M.D et al. (2008) General and Abdominal Adiposity and Risk of Death in Europe. The New England Journal of Medicine. 359:2105-2120

4. Scarborough, P. The economic burden of ill health due to diet, physical inactivity, smoking, alcohol and obesity in the UK: an update to 2006–07 NHS costs. Journal of Public Health. May 2011, 1-9

5. Childhood obesity: a plan for action. Published 18 August 2016.https://www.gov.uk/government/publications/childhood-obesity-a-plan-for-action/childhood-obesity-a-plan-for-action. Last accessed 21st September 2016

6. Obesity in Children. BMJ Best Practice. Feb 19 2016. http://bestpractice.bmj.com/best-practice/monograph/1085.html Last accessed 21st September 2016

7. Halvorsen JA, Vleugels RA, Bjertness E, Lien L. A population-based study of acne and body mass index in adolescents. Archives of dermatology. 2012 Jan 1;148(1):131-2

8. Egan K, Ettinger A, Bracken M. Childhood body mass index and subsequent physician-diagnosed asthma: a systematic review and meta-analysis of prospective cohort studies. BMC Pediatrics 2013;13(1):121

9. Black MH, Zhou H, Takayanagi M, Jacobsen SJ, Koebnick C. Increased Asthma Risk and Asthma-Related Health Care Complications Associated with Childhood Obesity. Am J Epidemiol 2013;6:6

10. Centre for Public Health Excellence at NICE (UK, National Collaborating Centre for Primary Care (UK. Obesity: the prevention, identification, assessment and management of overweight and obesity in adults and children

Chapter 35: Tired, temperature and a murmur
Dr Hugh Bishop

(35)

Chloe, a 3 year old girl presents to her local district general paediatric department with a 2-week history of increasing tiredness. Three days ago she developed a limp and on the day of presentation she has developed spontaneous bruises on her abdomen, back, arms and legs. Her parents feel that she is clingy and not her normal self. She has no significant past medical history. On examination she is pale, with warm peripheries, and a 2/6 systolic murmur is noted, loudest at the upper left sternal edge. Her temperature is 37.6°C, her heart rate is 110/minute and she has a normal blood pressure. There is no respiratory distress and her chest is clear. She has a 3 cm liver edge and a 2 cm splenic edge palpable. Her abdomen is soft and is not tender.

Initial blood results are as follows:

Sodium	136 mmol/l	Haemoglobin	65 g/l
Potassium	3.8 mmol/l	White cell count	53 x 10^9/l
Urea	6.5 mmol/l	Platelets	24 10^9/
LDH	450 U/l		
AST	32 U/l		
ALT	28 U/l		
Albumin	34 g/l		
Chloride	111 mmol/l		

Q1. What is the most likely underlying diagnosis?

A.   Acute Lymphoblastic Leukaemia
B.   Acute Myeloid Leukaemia
C.   Idiopathic Thrombocytopaenic Purpura
D.   Neuroblastoma
E.   Non-accidental injury

Q2. Which investigation is most important prior to transfer to the regional children's hospital?

A.   Abdominal ultrasound scan
B.   Blood film
C.   Bone marrow aspirate
D.   Chest x-ray
E.   Serum urate

Q3. Which treatment is it most important to commence prior to transfer to the regional children's hospital?

A.   Blood transfusion
B.   Intravenous antibiotics
C.   Intravenous hyperhydration
D.   Oral Dexamethasone
E.   Platelet transfusion

Answers and Rationale

Q1.   **A: Acute Lymphoblastic Leukaemia**
Q2.   **D: Chest x-ray**
Q3.   **C: Intravenous hyperhydration**

Childhood malignancy is rare, affecting around 1 in 700 children from birth to 14 years of age. This equates to around 1500 new diagnoses per year in the UK. An average GP will see a single newly presenting childhood malignancy in the course of their career. Despite this, cancer is the leading disease related cause of death in children. The early recognition of symptoms suggestive of malignancy is vital to the timely diagnosis and treatment of these life threatening conditions, and all healthcare professionals who look after children should develop an understanding of the common presentations of the commonest childhood tumours, and should know the early steps in management, focussed on maintaining the safety of the child. Childhood cancer requires specialist care in a small number of specialist centres, but many patients initially present to their GP, emergency department or their local DGH paediatric department. There is a balance to be struck between timely transfer to specialist care and immediate emergency investigation and management to maximise the safety of the child.

Any of the diagnoses in question 1 are possible, but the presence of hepatosplenomegaly combined with a short history make a new malignancy most likely. Splenomegaly and a raised white blood count would be unusual in neuroblastoma, and in this age group, acute lymphoblastic leukaemia is the commonest malignancy, and is considerably more common than acute myeloid leukaemia. While ITP does not cause hepatosplenomegaly, some of the viral infections that trigger it could, but the presence of anaemia and a raised white cell count make this unlikely. It is important to remember that even in the presence of a medical explanation for an increased bleeding tendency, that non-accidental injury may occur, and the pattern of any bruising should always be consistent with the explanation given before it can be discounted.

All of the investigations listed in question 2 will be performed, but when facing a question like this, it is vital that you pay attention to the wording of the question. A blood film is a quick and easy test, which can be done in any haematology lab, and it may confirm a diagnosis, but it will not have an impact on the safety of the patient during. A bone marrow aspirate might be possible, particularly in a large DGH department which provides a shared care oncology service, and again will secure a diagnosis, but it would lead to an unnecessary delay in transfer to specialist care which may put the patient at risk. Serum urate is a useful investigation, and will help to judge the risk of tumour lysis syndrome (see Chapter 38), which is an important complication of malignancy. However, tumour lysis is usually precipitated by treatment of the underlying malignancy and is rarely spontaneous. Abdominal ultrasound will provide useful information about the hepatosplenic infiltration, but this has no bearing on the immediate safety of the child. A chest X Ray will identify possible mediastinal lymphadenopathy, which can present a threat to the patient's airway, and is therefore vital to exclude prior to transferring the patient, and will guide the type of transfer, be it parental, by ambulance, or a PICU retrieval. This question highlights the importance of pausing to reflect on the question being asked, as sometimes the correct answer is not the most obvious one.

Of the different treatment options listed, all are likely to be required. Impaired neutrophil function is a consequence of both malignancy and its treatment, but at the moment, there are no features to suggest infection, and therefore antibiotics are not the immediate priority. Tumour lysis syndrome (TLS) is a potentially life threatening complication of newly presenting malignancy, and particularly of its treatment. A raised white cell count and LDH are risk factors for TLS, and the immediate commencement of hyperhydration with clear fluids with no additional potassium is an important step to take pending transfer to specialist care.

This is often done in conjunction with medication to reduce uric acid load, such as allopurinol or rasburicase. Blood transfusion should be approached with caution, particularly in a patient with a high white cell count, as the viscosity of the blood will already be raised, and packed red cells will exacerbate this, risking leucostasis and end organ thomboses. Platelet transfusion is less of a risk to the patient, but the point highlighted here is that patients will often tolerate a very low platelet count without bleeding, and in the absence of haemorrhage, the decision to transfuse can be left until the patient is under the care of the specialist team.

Dexamethasone is a vital part of the initial treatment of acute lymphoblastic leukaemia, but should not be started until the patient has been pre-treated with hyperhydration, to minimise the risk of tumour lysis syndrome. It should also not be commenced until the definitive diagnostic investigations have been performed, as a rapid response to steroid may interfere with the accurate evaluation of the extent of the disease, for example complicating the identification of central nervous system involvement.

Syllabus Mapping

Cardiology

- Know the causes of murmurs palpitations, syncope and chest pain, understand the principles of management and know when to refer

Haematology and Oncology

- Know the causes and presentations of anaemia and their initial investigation and management

- Know and understand safe transfusion practice

- Know the causes of bleeding, purpura and bruising and recognise features in the presentation which suggest serious underlying pathology

- Know how to interpret haematological investigations including full blood count, blood film and coagulation studies

- Know the clinical manifestations of acute leukaemia, lymphoma, and solid tumours

- Understand the role of different health care professionals in shared care for oncological conditions

References and Further Reading

1. Stevens, Caron and Biondi, Cancer In Children, Clinical Management 6th Edition. Oxford University Press, 2012. ISBN 978-0-19-959941-7

2. Pizzo and Poplack. Lipincott Williams and Wilkins, Principles and Practice of Pediatric Oncology 7th Edition. 2015. ISBN 978-1451194234

3. Scheinemann and Boyce, Emergencies in Pediatric Oncology. Springer, 2011. ISBN 978-1461411734

Chapter 36: Still jaundiced....
Dr Nilesh Agrawal and Dr Mithilesh Lal

36

Max is a full term male infant with a birth weight of 3388 grams who was noted to have continuing jaundice on day 19 of life. He was born via a normal vaginal delivery to a primiparous Caucasian mother whose blood group is O+. Maternal records do not indicate any antenatal problems and he received intramuscular vitamin K at birth.

Jaundice was first reported by midwives on day 5 when the newborn blood spot screening was performed. He was said to be breast feeding well and his current weight is 3600 grams.On examination his temperature is 36.7⁰C, heart rate 130/minute, and respiratory rate 40/minute. He appears well, with visible jaundice of his skin and conjunctiva. His liver was just palpable, but there was no splenomegaly.

Q1. Which one of the following would make you concerned about serious liver disease?

A.   Antenatal history of oligohydramnios
B.   Maternal history of hypothyroidism
C.   Maternal history of alcohol misuse in pregnancy
D.   History of pale stools and dark urine
E.   History of poor feeding and weight gain

Blood tests are taken and the initial results are:

Haemoglobin	103 g/l	Serum bilirubin	232 micromol/l
Packed cell volume	58%	Conjugated bilirubin	6 micromol/l
White blood count	20.9 x 10⁹/l	Albumin	25 g/l
Platelets	257 x 10⁹/l	ALP	250 U/l
		ALT	35 U/l

Q2. Which one of the following investigations should you request next?

A.   α1-antitrypsin levels
B.   Blood culture
C.   Liver ultrasound scan
D.   Thyroid function test
E.   Urine microscopy and culture

Q3. What is the most likely diagnosis?

A.   ABO/Rh incompatibility
B.   Biliary Atresia
C.   Breastmilk jaundice
D.   Congenital CMV infection
E.   Hereditary spherocytosis

Answers and Rationale

Q1. **D: History of pale stools and dark urine**
Q2. **E: Urine microscopy and culture**
Q3. **C: Breastmilk jaundice**

Jaundice is common in newborn infants. Approximately 60% of term and 80% of preterm babies develop jaundice in the first week of life, and about 10% of breastfed babies are still jaundiced at 1 month of age (1). In most babies early jaundice is usually harmless (often termed 'physiological jaundice'). However, a few babies will develop severe jaundice and its complications including bilirubin encephalopathy (kernicterus) if untreated. Box 36.1 lists factors that indicate pathological jaundice in infants.

• Early onset of clinical jaundice in the first 24 hours of age
• Rapid rise of serum bilirubin >100 micromol/l/24 h
• Sick newborn with jaundice
• Serum bilirubin >250 µmol/l by 48 h of age or >300 µmol/l by 72 h of age
• Failure to respond to phototherapy
• Prolonged jaundice - >14 d in term infants and >21d in preterm infants
• Conjugated bilirubin level of >35 µmol/l
• Pale chalky stools and dark urine

Box 36.1: Indicators of pathological jaundice in newborn infants

The baby in this scenario has prolonged jaundice. Prolonged jaundice is defined as jaundice persisting beyond the first 14 days in term infants and 21 days in preterm infants. Screening investigations for prolonged jaundice are listed in (Box 36.2).

• Conjugated and total serum bilirubin
• Full blood count and blood film (features of haemolysis)
• Blood group and direct antiglobulin test
• Thyroid function tests
• Urine microscopy and culture
• Urine for reducing substances
• Liver function tests

Box 36.2: Screening investigations for prolonged jaundice in neonates

It is important to differentiate between conjugated and unconjugated jaundice as the underlying diagnosis for each will be different. Understanding the physiology of bilirubin production will help you understand the potential causes of both conjugated and unconjugated jaundice. Bilirubin is mainly produced from the breakdown of red blood cells. Red cell breakdown produces unconjugated bilirubin, which circulates mostly bound to albumin although some is 'free' and hence able to enter the brain. Unconjugated bilirubin is metabolised in the liver to produce conjugated bilirubin which then passes into the gut and is largely excreted in stool, with a smaller amount being re-absorbed in the enterohepatic circulation.

This baby has unconjugated hyperbilirubinaemia. NICE guidelines provide recommendations for the investigation and management of jaundice in babies, (box 36.3) with this baby needing to have thyroid function tests, urine microscopy, urine culture and urine reducing substances to complete the initial prolonged jaundice screen. The clinical history tells you that the newborn screening blood spot has been performed and therefore the babies TSH level will have been assessed at that point. Whilst TFTs are still indicated the diagnosis of hypothyroidism is unlikely. Urinary tract infections are a relatively common cause of prolonged jaundice and therefore microscopy and culture is indicated. Reducing substances should also be tested for, but a metabolic diagnosis is much less likely than a Urinary tract infection (UTI).

- Haemolysis due to Rhesus, ABO or other isoimmunisation, heriditary spherocytosis and other red cell morphological abnormalities, Enzyme deficiency (G6PD, pyruvate kinase)
- Breast milk jaundice
- Infections including UTI
- Endocrine conditions e.g. hypothyroidism, hypopituitarism
- Metabolic causes e.g. glucuronyl transferase deficiency, galactosaemia

Box 36.3: Common causes of prolonged unconjugated jaundice

Breastfed babies are more likely than formula-fed babies to develop jaundice, both within the first week of life as well as beyond 2 to 3 weeks of age. Early jaundice in breastfed babies is thought to be due to a combination of factors, such as dehydration, poor gut motility, failure to pass meconium – all of which tend to cause increased enterohepatic circulation of bilirubin. These factors in isolation or in combination may also have a role in "breast milk" jaundice later.

Breast milk jaundice presenting as prolonged jaundice is seen in well babies who are thriving, have normal clinical examination apart from clinical jaundice and there is no evidence of haemolysis or infection. Parents should be reassured and breastfeeding continued. Pregnanediol metabolite or esterified fatty acids in breast milk may have inhibitory effect on hepatic conjugation through UGT enzymes. Alternatively, this may increase β-glucuronidase activity and deconjugate bilirubin, increase enterohepatic circulation of bilirubin and increase hepatic bilirubin load. These plausible mechanisms still remain unproven.

Jaundice from other causes may have to be ruled out, including blood group incompatibility (most commonly Rhesus or ABO incompatibility), other causes of haemolysis (breaking down of red blood cells), sepsis (infection), liver disease, bruising and metabolic disorders. Deficiency of a particular enzyme, glucose-6-phosphate-dehydrogenase, can cause severe neonatal jaundice. Glucose-6-phosphate-dehydrogenase deficiency is more common in certain geographical/ethnic group (eg Mediterannean and African).

Prolonged conjugated hyperbilirubinaemia is less common. The main causes are listed in box 36.4. An important diagnosis to make in these babies is biliary atresia as the outcome is much better if this condition can be operated on before 8 weeks of age. Abdominal US scan and radioisotope scan (HIDA) are undertaken to confirm this diagnosis prior to referral to one of the specialist liver services in the UK.

- Intrauterine infections – TORCH
- Neonatal hepatitis
- Biliary atresia
- Choledochal cyst
- Parenteral nutrition related
- Metabolic e.g. cystic fibrosis, α1-antitrypsin deficiency, galactosaemia
- Intrahepatic cholestasis – syndromic and familial

Box 36.4: Common causes of prolonged conjugated jaundice

Syllabus Mapping

Neonatology

- Be able to recognise and initiate the management of common disorders in the newborn including sepsis

- Understand the causes and features of neonatal jaundice knowing when to refer for further investigation and be able to recognise early presentation of neonatal hepatitis and biliary atresia

References

1. NICE guidelines, Jaundice in newborn babies under 28 days; [CG98] Published date: May 2010

Further Reading

Ives NK. Neonatal Jaundice. In: Rennie JM (ed). Rennie and Robertson's Textbook of Neonatology. 5th ed. Churchill Livingstone Elsevier: 2012. P672-92

Kaplan M, Wong RJ, Sibley E, Stevenson D. Neonatal Jaundice and Liver Diseases. In: Martin RJ, Fanaroff AA, Walsh MC (eds). Fanaroff and Martin's Neonatal-Perinatal Medicine: Diseases of the Fetus and Infant. 10th ed. Elsevier Saunders: 2015. P1618-75

Chapter 37: The history helps
Dr Rebecca Kettle and Dr Chris Dewhurst

37

Jill, a 7 month old girl presents to her GP with difficulty in passing stools. Her mother describes her as not opening her bowels for 4-5 days at a time and when she does she passes a large, solid stool which is painful for her. She was breastfed until 6 months of age and has only ever opened her bowels 2-3 times each week and vomits infrequently. She appears to be in discomfort when passing stool.

On examination her abdomen is soft, non-tender with a palpable mass in the left iliac fossa. She has normal bowel sounds.

Q1. When managing a child with idiopathic chronic constipation who is impacted, which of the following is the best first management step?

A. Dietary advice and dietician referral
B. Macrogol disimpaction regime starting at high dose and reducing according to response
C. Macrogol disimpaction regime starting with low dose and increasing according to response
D. Regular lactulose
E. Regular macrogol laxative

She returns 1 month later and her symptoms remain. On occasions there has been bright red blood in her nappy following passing a stool. At this visit Jill's mother has brought her "Red Book" (Child Health Record) with her. This records that at birth Jill weighed 3.5 kg (50th centile) and when weighed last week her weight was on the 9th centile. Her newborn examination demonstrated a clicky right hip but nil else. She was discharged at 12 hours of life and the midwife check at home records that she passed meconium for the first time on day 3 of life.

Examination findings were the same as previous however on external inspection a small anal fissure is noted.

Q2. Which is the most concerning sign/symptom of her presentation?

A. Abdominal mass
B. Anal fissure
C. Blood PR
D. Failure to pass meconium within 48 hours of birth
E. Faltering growth

Q3. What diagnostic investigation is required?

A. Abdominal radiograph
B. Anorectal manometry
C. Contrast enema
D. Digital rectal examination
E. Rectal biopsy

Answers and Rationale

Q1.   **C: Macrogol disimpaction regime starting with low dose and increasing according to response**
Q2.   **D: Failure to pass meconium within 48 hours of birth**
Q3.   **E: Rectal biopsy**

This question addresses the common problem of childhood constipation. It is an important problem which can cause distress to the child and family alike which is why early, appropriate management is vital.

Addressing the problem of childhood constipation starts with a thorough history. In the first part of this question the child presents with an extremely common presentation, however important information in the history was not elucidated, in particular the passage of meconium in the neonatal period.

The initial information provided points to Jill presenting with idiopathic constipation and impaction. NICE guidelines provide clear guidance on how to investigate and manage idiopathic childhood constipation (1). Firstly, you need to determine if the child is impacted which is indicated by the presence of overflow soiling or a palpable faecal mass. If there is impaction, it is necessary to disimpact prior to commencing maintenance therapy.

The first line of disimpaction is with polyethylene glycol 3350 + electrolytes, starting with low doses and increasing depending upon the response. Sometimes this can cause an increase in overflow soiling and abdominal pain. Stimulant and osmotic laxatives may also be required if disimapction is unsuccessful using polyethylene glycol 3350 alone. Maintenance treatment is required once disimpacted, or for the treatment of constipation without disimpaction. Low dose of polyethylene glycol is the first line of treatment with stimulant or osmotic laxatives used as additional therapy if this fails. It may take several months for a regular bowel habit to be established and when this does happen the medication should be continued for several more weeks before being weaned off the medication. Children who are toilet training should remain on laxatives until toilet training is well established. Some children require laxative therapy for several years.

As well as medical management, it is important to focus on diet and behaviour management. Ensure a balanced diet and sufficient fluids are consumed. Foods high in fibre are recommended along with sufficient quantities of water. Behavioural interventions suited to the child or young person's stage of development and include scheduled toileting and support to establish a regular bowel habit, maintenance and discussion of a bowel diary and use of encouragement and rewards systems.

When Jill returns to her GP a more through history is obtained. The most concerning feature or 'red-flag' symptom is the failure to pass meconium within 48 hours of birth; the other features which should alert you to a non-idiopathic cause are the faltering growth and the history of constipation since birth (only passing stools 2-3 times per week).

Red flag symptoms to be aware of in taking a history of childhood constipation include (1):

- Timing of onset of constipation – reported from birth or first few weeks of life
- Passage of meconium - failure to pass meconium / delay (more than 48 hours in a term baby)
- Stool pattern – ribbon type stools (more likely in child under 1 year)
- Motor problems – leg muscle weakness, gross motor delay
- Abdominal distension with vomiting

During a history taking should any of the above factors be present the child should not be treated but referred to the appropriate specialist for further investigation. Similarly to history taking there are also a number of red-flag signs which may be present on examination of the child, including:

- Abnormal appearance (including bruising or multiple fissures, position/patency of anus)
- Gross abdominal distension
- Abnormal asymmetry or flattening of gluteal muscles, evidence of sacral agenesis, discoloured skin, naevi or sinus, hairy patch, lipoma, central pit (dimple that you can't see the bottom of), scoliosis
- Lower limb abnormalities – e.g. talipes, abnormal neuromuscular signs
- Abnormal reflexes

Failure to pass meconium within the first 24 hours of life is abnormal and 99% of term infants will pass meconium within 48 hours. Failure to pass meconium is indicative of a possible anatomic or neuromusculardisorder, most commonly Hirschsprung's disease. Other causes include meconium ileus (the presenting feature in 10% of children with cystic fibrosis), malroation +/- volvulus (when bilious vomiting is present), anorectal malformations and bowel atresia/obstruction.

Hirschsprung's disease is caused by the congenital absence of ganglion cells in the submucosal and myenteric plexus. The affected segment of bowel is in a constant state of spasm and unable to relax, resulting in a functional distal bowel obstruction. The aganglionosis begins at the anus and extends proximally for a variable distance, usually to the sigmoid colon but sometimes to the ascending colon and rarely can affect the whole large and small bowel. It most commonly presents in the neonatal period with delayed or failure of passage of meconium though can present later, as in Jill's case, with chronic constipation and failure to thrive. Abdominal x-rays will show gaseous distension but these are not diagnostic. Contrast studies will show the constricted bowel and the distended colon proximal to it. However a rectal suction biopsy is required to demonstrate the absence of ganglion cells. Management includes decrompessing the bowel daily with saline enemas or with formation of a colostomy and pulling the ganglionic bowel to be attached to the anus at a later stage. Diarrhoea and soiling can occur in the long term (2).

When approaching a question regarding a diagnostic investigation the key is to think whether the investigation will give you a diagnosis? Certain investigations may be appropriate, first line or provide supportive evidence but will they actually diagnose the underlying problem.

The basic rule for digital rectal examination (DRE) in children is – don't do it! Having said that; DRE is performed, occasionally but should only be done in specific situations by an experienced healthcare professional who can interpret the results. Anorectal manometry may demonstrate failure of the anal sphincter to relax upon rectal distension in Hirschsprung's disease, however it is not recommended in children.

Syllabus Mapping

Gastroenterology and Hepatology

- Know how to diagnose and manage constipation

Neonatology

- Know about common minor congenital abnormalities and their initial management

- Know about the identification, initial management and appropriate referral pathways for neonatal surgical problems including NEC

References and Further Reading

1. NICE guidelines, Constipation in children and young people: diagnosis and management [CG99] Published date: May 2010

2. John Wiley & Sons, Chapter 7 Bowel Obstruction in Jones' Clinical Paediatric Surgery. 31 Oct 2014

Chapter 38: Hot and miserable
Dr Hugh Bishop

38

Dougie, a 4 year old boy presents to the emergency department with a 3-day history of irritability and fever. On the day of presentation he is reluctant to walk, and has developed a distended abdomen.

On examination he is miserable and clingy to his father. He is pale and has a distended abdomen with a large mass palpable in the right upper quadrant. He has clinical signs of ascites and a right sided pleural effusion. He complains of pain on movement of his lower limbs and will not weight bear. His heart rate is 120/minute, blood pressure 150/90 mmHg, and his respiratory rate is 30/minute.

Initial blood tests are as follows:

Sodium	137 mmol/l	Haemoglobin	97 g/l
Urea	3.8 mmol/l	White cell count	4.2×10^9/l
Potassium	4.8 mmo/l	Platelets	396×10^9/l
Creatinine	48 µmol/l		
Chloride	105 mmol/l		
AST	48 U/l		
ALT	34 U/l		
Albumin	26 g/l		

Q1. Which one of the following investigations is most likely to establish a diagnosis?

A. Alfafetoprotein
B. Ferritin
C. Lactate dehydrogenase
D. Neurone Specific Enolase
E. Urine catecholemines

Q2. What is the most likely diagnosis?

A. Acute Lymphoblastic Leukaemia
B. Hepatoblastoma
C. Neuroblastoma
D. Non-Hodgkin Lymphoma
E. Wilm's Tumour

Q3. What is the most important initial therapeutic step?

A. Emergency chemotherapy
B. Emergency radiotherapy
C Intravenous hyperhydration
D. Intravenous morphine
E. Laparotomy to remove the tumour

Answers and Rationale

Q1.   **E: Urine catecholemines**
Q2.   **C: Neuroblastoma**
Q3.   **D: Intravenous morphine**

It should be obvious to any paediatric trainee doctor that Dougie has a serious underlying pathological diagnosis and given the nature of presentation, with abdominal mass, hypertension and free fluid in the abdomen and chest, the most likely pathology is a malignant one. When faced with a question like this, or indeed in clinical practice with a patient like this, it is important to approach the diagnosis, investigation and management in a logical manner, informed by an understanding of the underlying epidemiology of childhood cancer, and always maintaining a focus on the emergency management of the patient during the diagnostic process.

In the first and second questions, regarding investigations most likely to establish a diagnosis and what that diagnosis is likely to be, you should think about which abdominal tumours may present in a child of this age. Neuroblastoma is the commonest non-central nervous system childhood solid tumour, but an abdominal mass could also be seen in hepatoblastoma, leukaemia, lymphoma, Wilm's tumour, or an array of other rare tumours such as germ cell tumours or soft tissue sarcomas.

Consider Dougie's clinical features of rapid presentation, hypertension, pain and misery. These are typical of high risk neuroblastoma, but not of the other most common solid abdominal tumours. Leukaemia and lymphoma are plausible, but the normal blood count and the large abdominal mass, combined with the other clinical features, especially hypertension, make these less likely. The mass and hypertension could be present in a Wilm's tumour, but in the absence of tumour rupture, pain is less common, and the bone pain suggested by reluctance to weight bear is not seen. Hepatoblastoma would fit with the location of the mass, but again the overall clinical picture of an acutely unwell child with irritability and pain are not classical, and in terms of epidemiology hepatoblastoma is significantly less common than neuroblastoma.

While it is vital to understand that the only investigation which will definitively establish a diagnosis is a biopsy of the tumour, there are many investigations that will be performed prior to this, which may strongly suggest one diagnosis over the others. All of the investigations listed in question 1 will be performed, but you must focus on the wording of the question, and judge which is most *likely* to establish the diagnosis.

LDH is a non-specific test, and may be raised in any malignancy. It is useful to know as it will guide your assessment of risk of tumour lysis syndrome. Tumour lysis syndrome is an oncological emergency (1), which results from the breakdown of dying tumour cells and the release of their intracellular contents in the form of purines and their breakdown products, ultimately uric acid, and electrolytes, particularly potassium and phosphate. Uric acid can be deposited in the renal tubules as urate crystals, leading to renal insufficiency, and the renal threshold for potassium and phosphate can be exceeded, leading to life threatening accumulation of these electrolytes. Phosphate ions can then bind with calcium to form calcium phosphate, which can also be deposited in crystalline form, further impairing renal function. Tumour lysis syndrome is most often precipitated by the treatment of cancer, particularly high grade B cell malignancies, or high white blood cell count leukaemia, but it can be present in any bulky tumour, and can occur spontaneously or in response to other physiological stressors such as anaesthesia or surgery.

Urine catecholemines measure the concentration of catecholemines, phenolic acids, and metadrenalines in the urine. These are hormones secreted by the sympathetic nervous system, and in neuroblastoma, an unregulated growth of cells with sympathetic nervous system origin, they will very commonly be abnormally raised, and in conjunction with this clinical presentation will make a diagnosis of neuroblastoma almost certain (but you still need a biopsy!).

Alfafetoprotein will be significantly raised in the majority of hepatoblastomas, and in secreting germ cell tumours, but will not distinguish between the two. Neurone specific enolase is an enzyme which can be over expressed by tumours whose embryological origin is the neural crest (including neuroblastoma), and if raised, it can be useful as a marker of response to treatment, and for future monitoring for tumour recurrence. However whilst it is often raised in neuroblastoma it is neither sensitive nor specific. Ferritin may be raised in any malignancy, and is of prognostic significance in neuroblastoma, but is not diagnostic of any individual tumour.

In any question about the initial management of a patient, take a step back and think about the patient in front of you. Do they have any compromise of airway, breathing or circulation? Are they in pain? Is there evidence of sepsis? It is easy to become fixated on the management of the underlying condition, but unless this is vital to ABC or relieving immediate distress, it is unlikely to be the correct answer. In the third question, any of the answers are plausible, but the absolute priority is to relieve the pain that is clearly described, and this should be with carefully titrated intravenous morphine.

Hyperhydration is used as part of the prophylaxis of tumour lysis syndrome. Its aim is to maintain good hydration and urine output to allow clearance of the toxic metabolites released from the dying tumour cells described earlier. It will be part of the early management of this patient, but bear in mind that tumour lysis syndrome is not common in most solid malignancies, and in the presence of ascites and pleural effusion, hyperhydration should not be rushed into without careful thought and involvement of both the oncology and renal teams.

Emergency chemotherapy is a possibility, and may help to control the ascites and pleural effusion, and subsequently improve the pain, but it is always going to take longer to organise than the simple measure of analgesia. Radiotherapy involves the use of ionising radiation delivered to the tumour, which disrupts the formation of new DNA by tumour cells, thereby impairing their ability to replicate. Emergency radiotherapy is rarely required, is not going to have an immediate effect, and is reserved for the control of life threatening symptoms where surgery may not be possible, and chemotherapy may be challenging to deliver, such as some cases of airway compromise, mediastinal compression or spinal cord compression from the tumour. Even emergency radiotherapy will require hours or days to organise and plan, and it is therefore unlikely to be the initial step in the management of any patient. In the case of tumour rupture or uncontrolled haemorrhage from the tumour, emergency surgery may be necessary, but this is a last resort, as the overall clinical state of the child will make it extremely risky.

Syllabus Mapping

Haematology and Oncology

- Know the causes of bleeding, purpura and bruising and recognise features in the presentation which suggest serious underlying pathology

- Know the clinical manifestations of acute leukaemia, lymphoma, and solid tumours

- Know how to assess a child with lymphadenopathy or other masses and when to refer

- Know about the risks and benefits of ionising radiation

References

1. Cairo MS, Bishop M. Tumour lysis syndrome: new therapeutic strategies and classification. British journal of haematology. 2004 Oct 1;127(1):3-11

Further Reading

Stevens, Caron and Biondi, Cancer In Children, Clinical Management 6th Edition. Oxford University Press, 2012. ISBN 978-0-19-959941-7

Pizzo and Poplack, Principles and Practice of Pediatric Oncology 7th Edition. Lipincott Williams and Wilkins, 2015. ISBN 978-1451194234

Scheinemann and Boyce, Emergencies in Pediatric Oncology. Springer, 2011. ISBN 978-1461411734

Chapter 39: Collapse at school
Dr Jill Spencer

Ceri is a 16 year old girl who is referred to from the emergency department after collapsing at school. On meeting her you note that she is very thin, with her height on the 75th centile and her weight on the 9th centile. She denies any recent weight loss. On examination her heart rate is 38/minute and axillary temperature is 36°C. She has dry hair and skin. Aside from being thin, you are unable to detect any other physical abnormalities. Her mother attends from work and confesses to you that she is concerned both about her daughter's weight loss and an apparent obsession with exercise.

Q1. Which one of the following is the most urgent investigation?

A.   ECG
B.   Full Blood Count
C.   Liver Function Tests
D.   Urea and Electrolytes
E.   Urinalysis

Q2. Which one of the following is the leading cause of death in people with anorexia nervosa?

A.   Cardiac Arrest
B.   Hypoglycaemia
C.   Liver Failure
D.   Sepsis
E.   Suicide

This is a list of potential diagnoses for adolescents presenting with weight loss:

A.   Anorexia Nervosa
B.   Bulimia Nervosa
C.   Chronic Fatigue Syndrome
D.   Coeliac Disease
E.   Crohn's Disease
F.   Depression
G.   Diabetes Mellitus
H.   Hyperthyroidism
I.   Juvenile idiopathic arthritis
J.   Ulcerative Colitis

For each of the following scenarios, choose the one most likely diagnosis.

Q3a. A 16 year old girl attends clinic with her father who is worried about her weight and persistent fatigue. On further questioning you discover that her periods have become irregular. On examination you note she has mouth ulcers and parotid gland enlargement. Her teeth are discoloured and she has a hoarse voice. She has discolouration over the metacarpalphalngeal joint of 3 fingers on her right hand. Blood gas analysis reveals a hypochloremic, hypokalemic metabolic alkalosis.

Q3b. A 13 year old boy presents with mouth ulcers. He complains of intermittent abdominal pain and occasion blood in his stools, and has lost weight in recent months. Laboratory tests reveal a microcytic anaemic with thrombocytosis and a raised ESR.

Q3C. A 15 year old girl presents with a 4-month history of tiredness and sleep disturbance, She was previously a high achiever, but admits to having difficulty concentrating at school and both her performance and attendance have been affected. She complains of dizziness and flu-like symptoms, but physical examination does not reveal any abnormality.

Answers and Rationale

Q1.   **A: ECG**
Q2.   **E: Suicide**
Q3a.   **B: Bulimia Nervosa**
Q3b.   **E: Crohn's Disease**
Q3c.   **C: Chronic Fatigue Syndrome**

The differential diagnosis of weight loss, particularly in teenagers is vast. Sudden and unintentional weight loss requires immediate assessment as it could represent a number of serious disease conditions. However, there is also an increased prevalence of psychological and social factors during pubertal years which influence the considerations of differential diagnoses. The approach to diagnosis requires a thorough medical history, but also an appreciation of the different perspectives and information gleamed from accompanying adults. At a time where teenagers are maturing and gaining increasing responsibility for their own health and decisions, the approach demands great sensitivity. This point is demonstrated in the initial scenario, where despite clear physical indicators, after collapsing at school Ceri denies recent weight loss; a fact that is contradicted by her mother.

Anorexia Nervosa typically has an onset in adolescence, affecting females predominantly. It is a clinical diagnosis, centred around significant weight loss resulting in extreme cachexia. Though patients often deny any associated symptoms, the condition gradually affects all the organ systems. Initial management is usually commenced in the community setting, but there are a number of indications for hospital admission. High risk cardiovascular features include: a heart rate less than 40 when awake, ECG evidence of biochemical abnormalities and a prolonged QT interval (1). The most important investigation therefore for Ceri is an ECG. The other investigations listed will be required but they are not as urgent as the ECG. Liver damage results from severe malnutrition evidenced by raised transaminases. The most common electrolyte abnormality is hypokalaemia however hyponatraemia may also result from excessive water ingestion. Urea and creatinine are usually low reflecting the inadequacy of nutrition. Whilst cardiac arrest is the most frequent *medical* cause of death among people with anorexia, there is a strong association with other mental health illnesses, and suicide remains the overall leading cause of death. Feeding is a treatment for anorexia and can be done against the will of the patient. Where there is refusal of treatment, consideration should be given to the application of the Mental Health Act 1983. Patients who are treated in this way require the input of both a Consultant Psychiatrist and a Consultant Paediatrician.

In question 3a, there are maternal concerns about weight loss once again, but there are physical elements that differentiate bulimia from anorexia. Bulimia is an eating disorder characterised by periods of excessive overeating or binging, followed by self-induced vomiting. It may also be associated with laxative abuse. Those who experience bulimia have a fear of gaining weight, but not all are under weight. Repeated vomiting erodes teeth enamel and leads to caries. Occasionally scarring or callouses can be apparent on the metacarpopharyngeal joints of the hand used to induce vomiting. This is called Russell's sign and occurs when the joints make contact with incisor teeth whilst inducing the gag reflex at the back of the throat. Parotid gland stimulation and enlargement occur in response to binge over-eating and excessive vomiting. The metabolic derangement that results is similar to that seen in other causes of persistent vomiting, such as pyloric stenosis. There is depletion of hydrogen ions and chloride ions from the stomach. In an attempt to maintain normal pH, the kidney retains hydrogen ions at the expense of potassium and gradually a hypochloraemic, hypokalaemic metabolic acidosis results.

Though there is a peak of eating disorders causing weight loss in adolescents consideration should neither be limited nor necessarily primarily focused on this. A range of important and serious alternatives may explain weight loss, and this is where a good history is critical. Pathological causes of weight loss can be broadly divided into inadequate intake, inadequate absorption or increased metabolic demands of an underlying medical condition.

In the scenario where a teenager presents with mouth ulcers and abdominal pain (Q3b.) the consideration should focus on intestinal diagnoses. Mouth ulcers, abdominal pain and bloody stools can be associated with Coeliac Disease (and this should be excluded by the investigation profile), but the accompanying blood picture in the 13 year old boy is suggestive of an inflammatory condition. Inflammatory Bowel Disease is characterised by inflammation and ulceration of the gastrointestinal tract leading to a variety of initial presentations and ongoing symptoms. Such presentations include faltering growth in younger children and weight loss in the adolescent population. A combination of different blood tests act as an initial screening tool. Thrombocytosis and microcytic anaemia are commonly found with both Crohn's Disease and Ulcerative Colitis. Other useful tests include CRP, ESR and Albumin. The absence of an abnormality with these parameters makes a diagnosis of IBD significantly less likely (2). A number of factors differentiate between the two conditions, with colonoscopy and examination of histological specimens key to accurate diagnosis, but the presence of aphthous ulceration is characteristic of Crohn's Disease.

Clinical assessment needs to include exclusion of other metabolic and endocrine disturbances, including blood glucose for the exclusion of Diabetes Mellitus and thyroid function test for the exclusion of hyperthyroidism, both of which are associated with weight loss. These investigations should be undertaken for the 15 year old girl in 3c, but it is unlikely that an abnormality would be found. There is an increasing recognition of the markers of Chronic Fatigue Syndrome; a complex condition characterised by persistent fatigue that limits an individual's ability to carry out ordinary activities, and is not diminished by sleep or rest. Chronic Fatigue Syndrome is associated with a range of other complaints including sleep disturbance, cognitive dysfunction and physical manifestations such as joint pain, headaches and dizziness. A diagnosis should only be made with the input of a Consultant Paediatrician when the symptoms have persisted for more than 3 months and other possible diagnoses have been excluded. The National Institute for Clinical Excellence (NICE) has released comprehension guidance relating to the diagnosis and management of this condition (3).

In summary, there are a number of factors to consider in an approach to investigation and management of a teenager with weight loss. Whilst considering physical diagnoses, it is important to retain awareness of the relationships between physical and mental health and be able to distinguish intentional from unintentional weight loss using history both the teenager and their guardians, an awareness of the physical manifestations of disorders of mental health, and how investigations can augment the approach to diagnosis and management.

Syllabus Mapping

Adolescent Health/Medicine

- Know how the health needs of adolescents are different from other age groups and about good practice in transition to adult services

- Know about the clinical presentation of young people with eating disorders

Behavioural Medicine/Psychiatry

- Know the determinants of child and adolescent mental health

- Know about the effects of physical disease on behaviour and vice versa including somatisation disorders

- Understand the principles of managing common emotional and behaviour problems such as temper tantrums, breath-holding attacks, sleep problems, feeding problems, the crying baby, oppositional behaviour, enuresis and encopresis, excessive water drinking, school refusal, bullying and chronic fatigue syndrome and know when to refer

- Know the features of depression in children and adolescents and when to refer to specialist services

Gastroenterology

- Know the presentations, causes and management of chronic and recurrent abdominal pain including when to refer

- Know the common causes of upper and lower gastrointestinal bleeding, initial management and appropriate referral

References and Further Reading

1. Royal College of Psychiatrists (2012a) Junior MARSIPAN: Management of Really Sick Patients under 18 with Anorexia Nervosa (CR168). Royal College of Psychiatrists

2. Cabrera-Abreu JC, Davies P, Matke Z, Murphy MS. Performance of blood tests in diagnosis of inflammatory bowel disease in a specialist clinic. Archives of Disease in Childhood. 2004;89:69-71

3. National Institute for Health and Clinical Excellence (2007).Chronic fatigue syndrome/myalgic encephalomyelitis (or encephalopathy): diagnosis and management. NICE guideline (CG53)

Chapter 40: A breathless baby
Dr Jill Spencer

You are asked to review a term baby boy, George, at 6-hours of age with grunting. He was born by spontaneous vaginal delivery following pre-labour rupture of membranes of 16 hours. At delivery he did not require any resuscitation and there were no immediate respiratory concerns. He fed well initially but his mum has struggled to feed him since then. On examination he has a loud expiratory grunt. His respiratory rate is 80/minute with subcostal and intercostal recession, and a heart rate of 170/minute. His temperature is 36.3°C and his peripheries are cool. His oxygen saturations are 89% in air, and air entry is equal bilaterally.

Q1. What investigation is most likely to guide immediate management?

A.   Blood Culture
B.   Blood Gas
C.   CRP
D.   Chest x-ray
E.   Echocardiogram

Q2. What is the most common organism in early neonatal infection?

A.   Candida
B.   Escherichia Coli
C.   Group A Streptococcus
D.   Group B Streptococcus Pseudomonas
E.   Pseudomonas

Below is a list of potential diagnoses for neonates with respiratory symptoms:

A.   Choanal Atresia
B.   Congenital Diaphragmatic Hernia
C.   Meconium Aspiration Syndrome
D.   Neonatal Abstinence Syndrome
E.   Pneumothorax

F.   Pulmonary Agenesis
G.   Respiratory Distress Syndrome
H.   Sepsis
I.   Tracheo-oesophageal Fistula
J.   Transient Tachypnoea of the Newborn

For each of the following scenarios, choose the most likely diagnosis:

Q3a. A 24 week baby is born by spontaneous onset of premature labour in a mother who colonised with Group B Streptococcus. There was no time for antenatal steroids. At delivery, is vigorous but her respiratory effort is intermittent and requires 80% oxygen to achieve adequate saturations for the baby.

Q3b. An 8-hour old baby born at 37 weeks with a birth weight of 2.1 kg has repeated episodes of cyanosis. His oxygen saturations are noted to improve when he cries during cannulation. He has a loud murmur on auscultation and you think his eyes are small.

Q3c. Whilst cannulating a 1-hour old baby with additional risk factors for neonatal infection, you note that he is cyanosed. On examination he has reduced breath sounds on the left side and his heart sounds are heard over the right hemithorax. His chest appears to be much larger than his abdomen.

Answers and Rationale

Q1.   **B: Blood Gas**
Q2.   **D: Group B Streptococcus**
Q3a.   **G: Respiratory Distress Syndrome**
Q3b.   **A: Choanal Atresia**
Q3c.   **B: Congenital Diaphragmatic Hernia**

Respiratory symptoms and signs are extremely common in the neonatal period. Whilst there is a sound physiological basis for some of these presentations representing the transition to ex-utero life, a wide range of differential diagnoses must be considered. Once any emergency steps have been taken to stabilise the baby, a thorough maternal history should be taken in order to identify any elements that may assist with diagnosis. A top-to-toe examination is indicated, even where the diagnosis seems straightforward, to ensure that other important abnormalities are not overlooked.

Group B streptococcus (GBS) is present as part of the normal gut flora in around one third of men and women, and colonises the vagina in around one quarter of all women. Half of babies born to mothers who are colonised be colonised themselves during delivery, but only 1 in 200 of these babies will develop GBS disease (1).

Pregnant women in the UK are not routinely screened for GBS carriage in pregnancy, but they may be investigated in pregnancy if they have symptoms of an infection. If GBS is detected on swabs or urine culture they will be offered prophylactic antibiotics following the onset of labour. Though GBS is the most common pathogen, other pathogens must be considered when targeting infection. Escherichia Coli is the second most common pathogen, and for this reason the choice of antibiotic should include Gram negative cover. Gentamicin is often used for this reason.

There are a number of situations in which the risks of GBS infection in the baby are increased, commonly referred to as 'risk factors for infection' and include (2):

- Invasive group B streptococcal infection in a previous baby
- Maternal group B streptococcal colonisation, bacteriuria or infection in the current pregnancy
- Prelabour rupture of membranes
- Preterm birth following spontaneous labour (before 37 weeks' gestation)
- Suspected or confirmed rupture of membranes for more than 18 hours in a preterm birth
- Intrapartum fever higher than 38°C, or confirmed or suspected chorioamnionitis
- Parenteral antibiotic treatment given to the woman for confirmed or suspected invasive bacterial infection (such as septicaemia) at any time during labour, or in the 24-hour periods before and after the birth (This does not refer to intrapartum antibiotic prophylaxis)
- Suspected or confirmed infection in another baby in the case of a multiple pregnancy

In the first scenario the baby had one known risk factor for infection (prelabour rupture of membranes). Where a single risk factor is present, it is common practice to observe the baby for signs of deterioration;

where two or more risk factors are present, the recommendation is that blood cultures are taken at birth and the baby is treated with antibiotics. (2) When there is a change in the clinical condition, even where there have been no risk factors, infection should be at the top of any list of differential diagnoses and investigations and management should be directed appropriately. In this baby the clinical presentation is highly suspicious for infection and a blood culture is the investigation most likely to aid diagnosis. However, it will take some time for this investigation to influence more specific management.

The first question specifically asks for the test which is most likely to guide immediate management and this is a blood gas. There are signs and symptoms of respiratory and cardiovascular compromise with low saturations, respiratory distress, tachycardia and poor perfusion. The information from a blood gas will help inform the need for respiratory support. It may also give an indication of the degree of circulatory compromise, from the base deficit and/or lactate, providing information about the possible need for a fluid bolus or inotropic support A chest x-ray is valuable in diagnosing a pneumothorax where there is clinical concern, but the presence of bilateral equal air entry makes this less likely in this scenario. A chest x-ray will form part of the investigations but should be prioritised after a blood gas. An initial CRP is most useful as a comparator with a measurement taken later in the episode. If two results taken 24 hours apart are 'negative' (the definition of which is dependent on individual laboratory values), bacterial infection is less likely; an initial low CRP is not sufficient to justify withholding antibiotic therapy (3). It is important to interpret these investigations in the context of the clinical presentation, using them to augment clinical decision-making, not to replace it.

In the other scenarios, infection should still be considered in the list of differential diagnoses, but there is other information to direct us towards alternative diagnoses. In question 3a, whilst infection may have triggered preterm labour in the mother of a 24-week baby, the gestation and lack of antenatal steroids make Respiratory Distress Syndrome, (also known as Surfactant Deficient Lung Disease) the most likely diagnosis for the respiratory presentation. The baby should also have blood cultures taken and receive treatment for a presumed infection, but a chest x-ray and the subsequent clinical course in response to surfactant administration will confirm this diagnosis.

In question 3b the 1-hour old baby is noted to be cyanosed except when he is crying. Though he should be treated for infection, this is an unusual pattern in conjunction with a heart murmur and the suggestion of dysmorphic features; thereby emphasising the importance of a full examination. The presence of cyanosis which improves with crying is classical for a presentation of choanal atresia. Given the presence of the heart murmur and small eyes, it is likely that this represents CHARGE association (see Chapter 30).

Part of the history in a sick neonate should always include consideration of antenatal scans. However, the presence of normal scans should be interpreted with caution; the timings of findings can be dependent on the severity of conditions and it is important to acknowledge that antenatal scans are screening examinations and not diagnostic. The baby in the final question has features that classically represent a congenital diaphragmatic hernia. Babies with congenital diaphragmatic hernias are usually diagnosed antenatally, but there are exceptions. This baby should still be treated for infection, but the clinical signs point towards a diagnosis of a left-sided diaphragmatic hernia. The care of this baby should quickly be escalated to the most senior level; these babies can deteriorate quickly and there is a high mortality associated with this condition.

In summary, the approach to the investigation, diagnosis and management of a neonate requires a systematic approach that begins with initial stabilisation followed by investigations targeted at the most likely diagnoses. Investigations should be used in conjunction with history and clinical examination to formulate a management plan that specifically addresses the clinical concerns.

Syllabus Mapping

Neonatology

- Know and understand the effects of antenatal and perinatal events

- Know the problems associated with prematurity and the long-term sequelae including the impact on the family and community

- Be able to recognise and initiate the management of common disorders in the newborn including sepsis

- Be aware of the occurrence and clinical features of maternal to fetal transmission of infection

- Know how to recognise, assess and initially manage respiratory disorders in the neonatal period

References and Further Reading

1. Benitz WE, Han MY, Madan A, Ramachandra P. Serial serum C-reactive protein levels in the diagnosis of neonatal infection. Pediatrics. 1998 Oct 1;102(4).

2. National Institute of Clinical Excellence. Neonatal infection (early onset): antibiotics for prevention and treatment. London: NICE; 2014

3. Group B Strep Support. (2016). Incidence of group B Strep infection in England, Wales & NI. Available at: http://gbss.org.uk/information-and-support/about-gbs/gbs-incidence/ (Accessed 6 Oct. 2016)

Chapter 41: Too small for rugby
Dr Priya Kumar

Matthew is a 13 year old boy who is referred to the general paediatric outpatient department by his GP as he is the smallest in his school year. He has not been selected for the school rugby team this year as his "too small". His mother reports that he eats well. He has had 1 episode of nocturnal enuresis. He opens his bowels 2 times per day and complains of occasional abdominal pain. He has been crying more frequently than usual and complains of joint pains. He was 4 kg born at term and fell to the 9th centile for weight at 6 months of age but returned to the 25th to 50th centile by 4 years of age.

On examination, he looks well. He has a few spots of acne on his back. His height is on the 9th centile and his weight is on the 50th Centile. Systemic examination is normal. His testes are 6 mls in volume with no penile enlargement (G2). He has adult type pubic hair confined to the pubis and adult type axillary hair. (A2, P2)

Q1. Which one of the following should be done first?

A.   Blood glucose measurement
B.   Body Mass Index
C.   Blood pressure measurement
D.   Calculate mid-parental height centile
E.   Urinalysis

Q2. What is the most important next investigation for Matthew?

A.   Bone age x-ray
B.   Calprotectin
C.   CRP
D.   Full blood count
E.   Thyroid function tests.

Q3. What is the next step of management?

A.   Reassure and discharge
B.   Refer to Endocrinologist
C.   Refer to Gastroenterologist
D.   Refer to Psychologist
E.   Review in 4 months

Answers and Rationale

Q1.   **D: Calculate mid-parental height centile**
Q2.   **D: Full blood count**
Q3.   **E: Review in 4 months**

Short stature is defined as height below 2 standard deviations of the mean for age. Common causes for short stature are listed in (box 41.1).

- **Normal variant** – familial or constitutional delay in growth and puberty
- **Endocrine** – hypothyroidism, hypopituitarism, growth hormone deficiency, Cushing's disease
- **Genetic** – Common cases are Noonan, Turner or Di George, Russel-silver syndrome but other genetic causes can cause short stature
- **Systemic disorders** – coeliac, inflammatory bowel or renal disease
- **Nutritional** – inadequate nutritional intake

Box 41.1: Common causes of short stature

Timely assessment is very important in children with short stature as if hormonal treatment is indicated by an underlying diagnosis it will only be effective before epiphyseal fusion occurs.

When faced with a child with short stature, the following "4 step approach" can be utilised for the identification of the underlying cause

1. Take accurate measurements of height and weight and refer to previous measurements from the child health record (known as "the red book"). Look at the growth velocity over infancy and childhood by reviewing previous height measurements over a 4 to 6 month period. Heights which have been continued on the same centile suggest a normal growth velocity Growth velocity determines the change in height over time. It is calculated as the difference in height on 2 different occasions annualised over a year (1).

2. Calculate the mid-parental centile:
    i.   Measure the height of both parents (cm)
    ii.   Add both heights together and divide by 2
    iii.   For boys, add 7 cm. For girls subtract 7 cm. this is the mid parental height
    iv.   Plot the mid parental height on a growth chart at the age of 18 years. This gives you the mid parental height centile. A normally growing child's height centile will be within two centile spaces (i.e. either one centile above or one centile below) of the mid-parental centile.

3. If short stature is confirmed (i.e below their genetic mid parental centile potential), look for other features including:

Weight
- If low, consider nutritional causes: malnutrition, bulimia, anorexia, chronic disease (causing malabsorption), psychosocial deprivation, neglect.
- If high, consider endocrine causes such as growth hormone deficiency or insensitvity, Cushing's syndrome, or hypothyroidism.

Height proportionality
- If sitting height and leg length disproportionate, consider a skeletal survey to identify limb and spinal causes of short stature e.g. achondroplasia, hypochondroplasia, conditions associated with spinal abnormalities or bone abnormalities e.g. rickets.
- If proportionate short stature, features may be present which suggest a specific syndrome and genetic testing or chromosome analysis would be warranted. Examples include Turner's, Noonan's, William's, Russell Silver syndrome, Prader Willi.

4. If the short stature does not fit into any of the above then it is likely due to constitutional delay of growth and puberty or familial short stature.

Constitutional delay of growth and puberty (CDGP) is suggested by deceleration of length/height in the first 3 years of life, a normal or near-normal height velocity during childhood (4–7 cm/year), with acceleration late in adolescence and the final adult height within the mid parental centile. Delayed bone age and pubertal development are also present. Questioning the parents about their childhood growth patterns and onset of puberty can help in the diagnosis as there is frequently a family history of similar growth patterns. Management includes reassurance and induction of puberty with Testosterone in some cases before epipyseal fusion. Although constitutional growth delay is a variant of normal growth rather than a disorder, delays in growth and sexual development may contribute to psychological difficulties, warranting treatment for some individuals (2).

Familial short stature can be characterized by early deceleration in linear growth depending on the infant's birth measurements, a normal or near-normal growth velocity in childhood, normal bone age and pubertal development, and height as an adult that is short, but appropriately within their genetic potential height centile.

In this case, Matthew's height is disproportionate to his weight. This may not be a problem if the mid parental height is within the 9th to 50th centile and hence this needs to be measured first. Children with familial short stature enter puberty at a normal time and typically complete growth with a height consistent with that of their genetic make-up from their parents. His weight is on the 50th centile so he is not overweight and therefore the Body mass index (BMI) is not the most important measurement. He has had only 1 episode of nocturnal enuresis and there are no other symptoms such as polyuria or polydipsia to suggest any glucose intolerance so testing the blood glucose level and urinalysis will not be the first choice investigations in elucidating the cause of his short stature. Blood pressure is always useful to identify whether there is an organic cause of short stature, but firstly we have to establish whether he is actually short compared to his genetic potential.

Anaemia due to chronic disease process such as inflammatory bowel disease, coeliac disease, renal disease can occur and these all contribute to short stature. Worldwide, malnutrition is the most common cause of growth failure and is usually related to poverty or anarchy. In developed countries, nutritional deficiencies are usually seen as a result of self-restricted diets (3). It should also be noted that neglect and psychosocial disturbances in a family can have an impact on a child's growth both in relation to height and weight.

Poor weight gain is often more noticeable than short stature. This is unlikely in this case as the boy's weight is on the 50th centile. CRP is increased in inflammatory cases such as Juvenile Chronic Arthritis and Calprotectin is raised in inflammatory bowel disease. The Thyroid function tests and bone age x-ray are all important tests to do as part of the investigative process of short stature but the full blood count to exclude anaemia should be the first test done to exclude any chronic disease which may be present and then other tests can be tailored to establish or exclude a potential cause of the anaemia if present.

Matthew is only 13 years old and is not yet established in puberty as indicated by his testicular volumes. Provided he has no underlying medical condition, he is likely to have constitutional delay in growth and puberty and hence should be reviewed to see whether he has further progressed in puberty and height. Regular monitoring of his height, weight, growth velocity and pubertal development over months or even years is required. Re-evaluation of the patient periodically is important to confirm the diagnosis and to monitor growth after the interventions have been made. Referral to colleagues can be instituted when a diagnosis is made of the cause of the short stature. Reassurance and discharge is not the correct option here as short stature has been linked to adverse psychological effects on teenage children and can be treated if an organic cause is found (2).

Syllabus mapping

Endocrinology and growth

- Understand the principles of and practice of growth measurement, including plotting and interpretation of growth charts

- Understand the patterns of normal growth and development including puberty and its normal variations

- Know the causes of abnormal growth including stature and slow or accelerated growth. Know about appropriate assessment, investigation and treatment

References

1. BMJ Best Practice. Assessment of short stature. Available at http://bestpractice.bmj.com/best-practice/monograph/749/diagnosis/step-by-step.html (last accessed 17th November 2016)

2. Quitmann JH, Bullinger M, Sommer R, Rohenkohl AC, Da Silva NM. Associations between Psychological Problems and Quality of Life in Pediatric Short Stature from Patients' and Parents' Perspectives. PloS one. 2016 Apr 20;11(4):e0153953

3. Kirby M, Danner E. Nutritional deficiencies in children on restricted diets. Pediatric Clinics of North America. 2009 Oct 31;56(5):1085-103

Further Reading

Cheetham T, Davies JH. Investigation and management of short stature. Archives of disease in childhood. 2014 Aug 1;99(8):767-71

Chapter 42: A 2 year old girl with delayed speech development
Dr Robert Dinwiddie and Dr Chris Dewhurst

42

Jyoti is a 2 year old girl, recently arrived from south Asia, who is referred to the GP by her health visitor with poor speech development. The referral letter includes the following:

"Jyoti makes some babbling sounds but has little understanding of words or simple commands. Her parents are also concerned that she is not hearing properly. On her 2 year developmental assessment her level of gross motor functioning was approximately 15 months. Her height and weight are on the 50th centiles and there are no dysmorphic features and physical examination is normal. She was born at term and received antibiotics for 7 days for possible sepsis. She did not have a neonatal hearing screening test."

Q1. Which one of the following tests would be most suitable to assess this girls hearing?

A. Automated auditory brainstem response
B. Automated otoacoustic emissions
C. Play audiometry
D. Speech perception test
E. Visual reinforcement audiometry

Q2. Which one of the following is the most likely cause of her hearing problem?

A. Antibiotic induced ototoxicity
B. Autosomal recessive hearing loss
C. Congenital Cytomegalovirus (cCMV) infection
D. Lack of stimulation
E. Waardenburg syndrome type 1

Q3. Which one of the following features would most strongly indicate that Jyoti was likely to have autism?

A. Being upset if separated from her favourite toy
B. Fascination with water
C. Having temper tantrums
D. Not making eye contact
E. Not obeying instructions

Answers and Rationale

Q1. **E: Visual reinforcement audiometry**
Q2. **C: Congenital Cytomegalovirus (cCMV) infection**
Q3. **D: Not making eye contact**

Jyoti has presented late due to the fact that she had lived abroad for the first 2 years of her life. If she had been born in the UK she would have had her hearing tested by the national Newborn Hearing Screening Programme. The majority of babies are tested within 48 hours of birth while still in hospital and the rest at home within the next few days. The standard test uses otoacoustic emissions (OAEs) which are sounds generated within the inner ear in response to an auditory stimulus. This is a reliable screening test for middle and inner ear hearing loss but does not test for abnormalities in the higher auditory pathways. Those who do not pass this screening test are referred for follow-up testing which utilises auditory brainstem responses (ABRs). This method will detect abnormalities throughout the entire hearing pathway (1). Other audiological tests used in the assessment of children are listed in (Table 42.1).

Test	When	How
Distraction test	Must be able to sit and turn the head to sound. 6 – 24 months	Requires 2 testers. The first tester maintains the child's attention through simple play. They then stop this distraction and the second tester positioned at 45 degrees behind the child presents an auditory stimulus which then varies in sound level and the side at which it is presented.
Visual Reinforcement audiometry	Must be able to sit and turn the head to sound. 6-30 months	Similar to the distraction test but the sound is played from speakers either side of the child. If they turn towards the sound a visual reinforcement (eg toy) is presented as a reward. The volume and pitch of the sound can then be varied.
Play audiometry	When able to follow simple commands, approx. 20 months – 5 years	The child is asked to perform a simple task (eg putting a toy in a basket) when sounds are played to the child through either through speakers or headphones.
Pure tone audiometry	When able to follow commands and understand instruction approx. 4 years +	Sounds at different volumes and frequencies are played and the child has to press a button after each sound.
Speech perception test	When there is a reasonable understanding of words. Age 3 years +	Assess the ability of the child to recognise words. The child will often have to point to a picture of the word being presented to them. It is important to ensure no visual clues are provided by making sure the child cannot see the testers lip movements.
Tympanometry	Any age	Assess the flexibility of the ear drum when air is applied at different air pressures. This is an assessment of middle ear function.

Table 42.1: Audiological tests performed in children

In a significant number of cases congenital hearing loss is genetically determined. Two major groups are described, those which are part of a syndrome (syndromic) and those in which it is an isolated finding on its own (non-syndromic). Several hundred syndromes with an associated loss of hearing have now been described as have more than 100 genes known to cause non-syndromic hearing loss. If there are no other abnormal features such as dysmorphism or an associated developmental delay, such as in this case, then the cause is likely to be due to an autosomal recessive genetic condition. In this situation the parents will have normal hearing but there is a high risk of recurrence in future siblings. A mutation in the gap junction beta-2 protein (GJP2) gene, also known as connexin 26 – Cx26, is the most common cause of congenital hearing loss in these cases. Congenital causes of sensorineural hearing loss are more common than those due to congenital Cytomegalovirus infection. In Jyoit's case however the presence of developmental delay makes Congenital Cytomegalovirus infection (cCMV) more likely.

Congenital CMV (cCMV) infection occurs in approximately 0.6% of pregnancies in developed countries. In the UK as many as 50% of pregnant women are seronegative (2). Although transmission occurs more frequently later in pregnancy, infection earlier in pregnancy carries a higher risk to the fetus. The rate of transmission is 30-40% in seronegative women but only 1% in those who have been infected previously (2). Approximately 10% of infants with cCMV have systemic symptoms and 60% of these have long-term neurological complications. Infants who are asymptomatic at birth have a 15% chance of developing sensorineural hearing loss (SNHL).

Confirmation of cCMV requires detection of CMV in body fluids within the first 3 weeks of life, saliva and urine samples carry the greatest diagnostic yield but neonatal blood spot tests can also be diagnostic. These tests utilise PCR to detect CMV viral DNA (2). Treatment of cCMV is most effective if started early during the first 4 weeks of life. Intravenous ganciclovir or oral valganciclovir are effective inhibitors of CMV replication. Careful monitoring for haematological and hepatological side effects is necessary. When Jyoti presents at the age of 2 years anti-viral treatment would be ineffective. Long-term audiological support and treatment would be necessary. At a later stage referral for a cochlear implant, which has been shown to be an effective treatment for cCMV infected patients may be necessary (1).

Jyoti also has a history of treatment for possible neonatal sepsis. In all probability this would have involved the administration of an aminoglycoside such as gentamicin. Ototoxicity due to exposure to aminoglycosides in the neonatal period is rare, and tends to result in high frequency hearing loss and is not usually as severe as in this case. The genetic mutation m1555A>G in mitochondrial RNA is known to increase the susceptibility to aminoglycoside induced ototoxicity (1).

The presence of motor delay means that cCMV is the most likely diagnosis as this would not be present if the cause was ototoxcity from aminoglycoside administration as a neonate.

Lack of stimulation, particularly lack of exposure to speech, is known to result in absence or severe delay in the onset of speech. This has to be extreme and is usually part of a much wider scenario of emotional and physical deprivation.

Waardenburg syndrome type 1 is an example of syndromic hearing loss. These children have bright blue eyes, hair between the eyebrows and widely spaced inner canthi of the eyes (1). The condition is inherited as an autosomal dominant and the diagnosis can be confirmed by the presence of a mutation in the PAX3 gene.

Autism is characterised by a qualitative impairmention in social interaction, communication and restricted, repetitive and stereotypical patterns of behaviour, interests and activities. It is a spectrum disorder and can present at any age. Features in toddlers can be wide and varied however common presentations include lack of speech, not responding to social clues (e.g not smiling in response to their parent smiling), lack of make believe play, not involving others in their world by pointing at objects, not being interested in other children, not copying parental behaviours and poor eye contact and repetitive 'stereotypical' movements such as hand flapping. The features listed in question 3 can all be part of normal toddler behaviour, however a lack of eye contact would be concerning regarding the development of autism and warrants further referral for a full multi-disciplinary assessment. This may include assessment by community paediatricians and/or child and/or adolescent psychiatrists, speech and language therapists and psychologists (3).

Syllabus Mapping

Neurodevelopment and Neurodisability

- Know the causes speech and language delay or disorder and principles of management including autism spectrum disorder.

Respiratory

- Recognise the presenting features of hearing impairment and principles of assessment and management

References

1. Rajput K, Bitner-Glindzicz M. Hearing and balance. In Science of Paediatrics MRCPCH Mastercourse. Eds Lissauer T, Carroll W. Elsevier, London 2017;ch31:609-626

2. Shah T, Luck S, Sharland M, Kadambari S, Heath P, Lyall H. Fifteen minute consultation: diagnosis and management of congenital CMV. Arch Dis Child Educ Prac Ed 2016;101:232-235

3. NICE guideline 128. Autism spectrum disorder in under 19s: recognition, referral and diagnosis. Published September 2011

Further reading

Goderis J, De Leenheer E, Smets K, Van Hoecke H, Keymeulen A, Dhooge I. Hearing loss in congenital CMV infection: a systematic review. Pediatrics 2014;134:972-982

Manicklal S, Emery VC, Lazzarrotto T, Boppana SB, Gupta RK. The silent global burden of congenital cytomegalovirus. Clin Microbiol Rev 2013;26:86-102

Chapter 43: A 15 Year old girl who has been to a party
Dr Robert Dinwiddie and Dr Chris Dewhurst

43

Sally is a 15 year old girl who attends the walk in center with a white, creamy vaginal discharge. She was initially reluctant to disclose any sexual activity but after further discussion she tells you that she had unprotected sex for the first time with her 16 year old boyfriend, 6 days previously at a party. She had planned to have sex with him that night and had drunk some alcohol at the party but denies being drunk when she had sex. Sally would like you to prescribe her the "morning after pill".

Sally asks you if it was legal to have consensual sex at her age.

Q1. Which one of the following is the best response to this question?

A.   It is illegal and the boy is likely to be prosecuted
B.   It is illegal and you have a duty to inform social services
C.   It is illegal however no further action will be taken
D.   It is legal as long as one partner is over 16
E.   It is legal as long as she was not drunk

Q2. Which one of the following is the next most useful test?

A.   Blood test for HIV serology
B.   Blood test for syphilis antibodies
C.   Pregnancy test
D.   Vaginal swab for culture
E.   Vaginal swab for nucleic acid amplification test (NAAT) for likely pathogens

Q3. Which of the following organisms is most likely to be the cause of her vaginal discharge?

A.   Candida albicans
B.   Chlamydia trachomatis
C.   Neisseria gonorrhoea
D.   Staphylococcus aureus
E.   Trichomonas vaginalis

Answers and Rationale

Q1.   **C: It is illegal however no further action will be taken**
Q2.   **E: Vaginal swab for nucleic acid amplification test (NAAT) for likely pathogens**
Q3.   **B: Chlamydia trachomatis**

Sally is displaying one of the major problems seen in adolescence, namely that of exploratory and risk taking behaviour. Adolescence is defined by the WHO as between the ages of 14 and 20 and this age group currently comprises 12.5% of the total population of the UK. Risk taking behaviours include, among others, smoking, drug and alcohol abuse and unprotected sex. The UK continues to have one of the highest rates of teenage pregnancies among western European countries. The median age of first heterosexual intercourse in the UK is currently 16 years (1, 2).

In the UK the age of consent for any form of sexual activity is 16. It is therefore an offence for anyone to have any sexual activity with a person under the age of 16. However, Home Office guidance is clear that children of the same or similar age are highly unlikely to be prosecuted for engaging in sexual activity, where the activity is mutually agreed and there is no abuse or exploitation (3). Specific laws protect children under the age of 13 who cannot legally give their consent to any form of sexual activity. It is important to be aware that there are different legal systems in England and Wales, Northern Ireland and Scotland. Often the laws are similar however there are subtle differences that paediatricians need to have knowledge of relating to consent for medical treatment, parental responsibility and consent to sexual activity.

In this case, Sally tells you that she has agreed to the sexual intercourse and that this was pre-planned, making exploitation or abuse unlikely. It would be important to ensure that she had fully agreed with having sex and that her boyfriend had not given her alcohol to compromise her decision making.

It is too late to administer the "morning after" pill as it only works for up to 120 hours after unprotected intercourse. Two preparations are currently available – levonelle, which works for up to 72 hours post coitus. It contains levonorgestrel, a progestogen which acts by thickening cervical mucus, inhibition of sperm survival and alteration of the endometrium which inhibits embryonic implantation. "EllaOne" is active for up 120 hours post intercourse and contains ulipristil acetate. This compound is a selective progesterone receptor modulator (SPRM) which results in delayed ovulation and endometrial maturation so inhibiting embryonic implantation. Young people over the age of 16 can obtain these over the counter and it is also licensed for those under 16 provided the pharmacist is satisfied that the young person requesting it fully understands the circumstances and the nature of what she is doing.

Six days after intercourse a pregnancy test would not yet be positive. This happens approximately 3-4 days after implantation of the fertilized egg. This would normally be 9 days after ovulation and fertilization which would coincide approximately with the date of the next menstrual period. If a pregnancy test were to be positive in this case it would indicate a pregnancy arising from previous sexual activity.

Given the vaginal discharge it is likely that Sally has a sexually transmitted infection. Chlamydia trachomatis is the most common sexually transmitted infection (STI) among adolescents in the UK. This age group also makes up the highest rate of new cases in the general population. Presentation with a post-coital discharge, as in this case, is typical. It can however be asymptomatic. If untreated it can result in long-term complications Including infertility, ectopic pregnancy and chronic pelvic inflammatory disease. Treatment is effective with a single dose of azithromycin.

Given that chlamydia is the most likely pathogen the most useful action in this case would be to send a nucleic acid amplification test (NAAT) for chlamydia (and also gonorrhoea). This test is performed on a urine sample, a vaginal swab (if necessary taken by the patient herself) or a blood sample. The test detects the presence of specific pathogens, including chlamydia or gonorrhoea, by the amplification of organism specific DNA. It becomes positive as soon as the organisms are present thus providing for rapid diagnosis and facilitating appropriate treatment. The test should be repeated 3 months after treatment is complete in order to ensure that this has been successful and to demonstrate that reinfection has not occurred.

In England since 2003 there has been a National Chlamydia Screening Programme (NCSP). Its objectives are to prevent and control chlamydia through early detection and treatment of infection, to reduce onward transmission to sexual partners, to prevent the consequences of untreated infection. Also to ensure that all sexually active under 25 year olds are informed about chlamydia, that they have access to sexual health services and to normalise the idea that regular chlamydia screening is an expected part of normal health care in this age group. People under 25 years can be tested by NCSP at pharmacies, contraception clinics or colleges with recommendations that you should get tested for chlamydia every year or when you change sexual partners (3). Similar initiatives have been established in Scotland and Northern Ireland.

Candida albicans is a much less common cause of STI. It is more prevalent in those who are immunosuppressed including patients on corticosteroids. When sexually transmitted it presents with itching, localised pain and inflammation in association with a vaginal discharge which may be thick and unpleasant smelling. Treatment is with a localised antifungal agent.

Gonorrhoea is the second most frequent STI in this age group (2). Although many cases are asymptomatic clinical presenting features include dysuria, urethral discharge, lower abdominal pain and inter-menstrual bleeding. Systemic symptoms can include photosensitivity, arthralgia, sore throat and lymphadenopathy. Long-term complications include chronic pelvic inflammatory disease, infertility and ectopic pregnancy. Treatment is with a single dose of a parenteral cephalosporin combined with oral azithromycin.

Staphylococcus aureus is a ubiquitous organism primarily resident on the skin. It is not infrequently grown from vaginal swabs but in otherwise healthy individuals it rarely causes problems if personal hygiene is maintained. The most serious complication is associated with tampon use. Toxin releasing staphylococci can flourish in this environment leading to the onset of toxic shock syndrome which is an extremely serious and often life-threatening condition. Treatment is with high dose intravenous anti-staphylococcal antibiotics and intensive life-support when necessary.

Trichomonas vaginalis is caused by a single cell anaerobic protozoan. It is a frequent but often unrecognised cause of STI. It is detectable on vaginal swabs. When symptomatic it results in localised genital inflammation, vaginal discharge, urinary frequency and dyspareunia. Treatment is with oral metronidazole. As with all STIs it is important that sexual partners are also screened and treated to prevent re-infection.

Although the incidence of chlamydia has fallen slightly in this age group in recent years that of syphilis has increased. Presentation is with a chancre, a painless ulceration visible in the affected area 3-4 weeks after primary infection. Syphilis antibodies initially become positive several weeks after primary infection so would not be useful in this case. The organism may however be visible on microscopy of a vaginal swab. Treatment is with penicillin.

Sending a vaginal swab for culture would be useful in the detection of each of the organisms described above. The NAAT test is however more immediately diagnostic for the detection of the most likely pathogen in this case.

Syllabus Mapping

Adolescent health

- Know about risk taking behaviours including non-adherence, deliberate self- harm and substance misuse and understand how these are managed within Health and Social Services

- Know about contraceptive and sexual health issues including sexually transmitted infections and teenage pregnancy and how to provide appropriate advice

Ethics and Law

- Understand the principles of child advocacy i.e. that all decisions are to be made in the best interests of the child and issues relating to consent and confidentiality.

References and Further Reading

1. Sargant NN, Hudson L, McDonagh J. Adolescent Medicine. In: The Science of Paediatrics. Eds Lissauer T, Carroll W. Elsevier, London 2017;ch32:627-639

2. Viner R. Adolescent Medicine. In: Training in Paediatrics. Eds: Gardiner M, Eisen S, Murphy C. Oxford University Press 2009;ch19:408-424

3. National Chlamydia Screening Programme. www.gov.uk/government/publications/ncsp-programme-overview

Chapter 44: Ophthalmology clinic
Dr Balamurugan Palanisami and
Dr Chris Dewhurst

44

You are working as an ST1 doctor in paediatrics and are revising for your MRPCH exams. You realise you know very little ophthalmology and that the theory examinations often contain ophthalmology questions. You therefore decide to go to the teaching hospital and observe a paediatric ophthalmology clinic.

The first child you see is a 3 year old boy, Tom, whose mum thinks he has a squint. Examination reveals normal ocular movements. Torch light test identifies convergent strabismus that becomes more exaggerated on accommodation. He is normally fit and healthy.

Q1. Which of the following is the most likely diagnosis?

A.   Abducens nerve (VI) palsy
B.   Downs Syndrome
C.   Hypermetropic refractive error
D.   Myopic refractive error
E.   Pseudo Squint

The second child is a 12 year old girl, Ciara, who presents with new onset of double vision. She has had mild headaches for the past couple of weeks that she has put down to exam stress. Examination of her eye reveals a left sided ptosis, dilated pupils and her left pupil is deviated inferiorly and laterally. She weighs 51 kgs (50th centile) and her height is 151 cms (9th centile)

Q2. Which of the following is the most likely diagnosis?

A.   Abducens nerve (VI) palsy
B.   Facial Nerve (VII) palsy
C.   Horner's Syndrome
D.   Oculomotor nerve (III) palsy
E.   Trochlear Nerve (IV) palsy

The third patient is a 2 day old boy, Jaxon, who has been referred by the paediatric team with absence of the red reflex in his left eye noted on his routine newborn examination. His birth weight was 3.2 kg and his head circumference 34 cm (both 25th centile). He also had a soft systolic murmur on his newborn check and will be reviewed with this in the outpatient's clinic in 6 weeks' time. His mother is 19 years old, is an ex-smoker and drank 2 glasses of wine per week whilst pregnant. She suffers with anxiety disorder and is severely needle phobic resulting in there being no booking blood results available.

Q3. Which of the following is the most likely diagnosis?

A.   Congenital Rubella syndrome
B.   Fetal alcohol syndrome
C.   Galactosemia
D.   Retinoblastoma
E.   Sporadic isolated cataract

Answers and Rationale

Q1.   **C: Hypermetropic refractive error**
Q2.   **D: Oculomotor nerve (III) palsy**
Q3.   **E: Sporadic isolated cataract**

There is limited exposure to ophthalmological problems in general paediatric training however it is important for you to be able to recognise, advise and refer appropriately the common ophthalmological problems. The children attending to the ophthalmology clinic are presenting with three relatively common problems; strabismus, ptosis and absent red reflex.

Strabismus

Strabismus (squint) occurs when one eye is misaligned with the other. It affects around 1 in 20 children and can occur at any age. Intermittent deviation of the eyes is common in healthy neonates before normal binocular co-ordination develops at around 3 months of age and should not cause concern in an otherwise healthy baby. Any strabismus after this age, or a constant squint in the first three months of life, warrants further evaluation.

A common presentation of strabismus is with the parent noticing that their child's eye is 'turning'. Sometimes the presence of a broad nasal bridge can give the appearance of a squint which on further testing demonstrates that the child does not have strabismus. This is termed pseudo squint.

When examining for strabismus it is important to classify using the following (1):

- **Direction of deviation.** Inwards (esotropia), outwards (exotropia), upwards (hypertropia) or downwards (hypotropia)

- **Deviation related to eye position.** With a concomitant strabismus the degree of deviation does not vary with the direction gaze. This is the most common strabismus and occurs as the balance between the muscles in the two eyes has been lost, there is no paralysis or limitation of eye movements. In a noncomitant strabismus the degree of deviation varies with the direction of gaze indicating an neurological or muscular disease causing paresis or paralysis of the extra-ocular muscles.

- **Latent or manifest.** A latent strabismus is present only when the use of both eyes is interrupted, for example, by covering one eye. A manifest strabismus is present when the eyes are open and being used so that when one eye views the object of interest the other eye is deviated. This may be constant, or intermittent.

- **Unilateral or alternating.** The strabismus may affect one eye only or alternate from eye to eye.

- **Relationship to accommodation.** An accommodative strabismus becomes exaggerated when accommodating and focusing on an object. The child is usually hypermetropic.

Strabismus' that give rise to concern about the underlying cause include constant unilateral exotropias, any acquired incomitant squint, and sudden, late onset (over 3-4 years) esotropia, all of which may indicate serious underlying brain pathology.

The commonest childhood strabismus in childhood is an accommodative esotropia which is usually seen in hypermetropia. Without glasses the image will naturally focus behind the retina but with accommodative effort the image can be forced to focus on the retina. This accommodative effort results in esotropia which will improve on wearing corrective glasses and sometimes cause complete resolution.

Any child who is detected to have a squint should be referred to the local paediatric eye service for full strabismus and visual acuity assessment by orthoptists. Management is directed to the underlying cause but may include corrective glasses, occlusion of the normal eye, surgery or botulinum toxin.

Ptosis

Ptosis refers to lowering of the upper eye lid lowering. The upper eye lid is elevated by the levator muscle which is innervated by the third (oculomotor) cranial nerve. Congenital ptosis is usually caused by a congenital disinsertion of the levator muscle. Surgery may be required to ensure normal visual development occurs. A rarer form of congenital ptosis is Marcus-Gunn 'jaw-winking' ptosis. This condition is usually first diagnosed in babies when the eye lid on one side rhythmically moves when feeding. It is thought to arise due to aberrant connections between the 5th (trigeminal) and 3rd cranial nerve. Usually no treatment is required.

Acquired forms of ptosis include conditions affecting either the nerve or muscle. The 3rd cranial nerve innervates most of the ocular movements and causes constriction and dilatation of the pupil. The 12 year old girl in question 2 has features indicating a 3rd nerve palsy. Common causes of a 3rd nerve palsy in children include trauma to the nerve from head injury, meningitis, compression of the nerve from a tumour or raised intracranial pressure or neurovascular compromise. Given the possibility of an intracranial mass lesion brain imaging would be the first investigation in this child has been performed.

Other causes of ptosis in children include neuroblastoma, Horner's syndrome or myasthenia gravis.

Absent Red Reflex

An absent red reflex (leukocoria) usually presents either at birth as part of the newborn check or in older children at opportunistic examinations. The classic story of a child whose auntie/grandfather/neighbour notices an abnormal "white eye" on flash photography occasionally occurs however the most common causes of this phenomenon include light being reflected off the optic nerve (which is white) and photographic angles that cause the light to be reflected in an unusual, asymmetric way between the two eyes (2). Nevertheless, a "white reflex" warrants further investigation with direct ophthalmoscopy because of the risk of serious underlying pathology. Children with darker skin tones may have pale retina and often visualisation of retinal vessels or comparing with the parents retina can provide reassurance. If uncertain, dilatation with cyclopentolate eye drops may help you see the retina.

Leukocoria evident on ophthalmoscopy result's from opacification of any of the structures through which light passes through on its way to the retina – the cornea, lens, vitreous and retina (3).

- **Cornea** – These are a rare cause of an absent red reflex but include mucopolysaccharidoses, cystinosis, fetal alcohol syndrome or corneal tears from forceps delivery.

- **Lens** - Cataracts are called "congenital" or "infantile" if they occur within the first year of life and "juvenile" if they occur in the first decade. Infantile cataracts may occur as a result of chromosomal anomalies, prenatal viral infections (eg TORCH; toxoplasmosis, rubella, cytomegalovirus and herpes simplex virus), metabolic conditions (e.g. galactosemia, homocystinuria), trauma and radiation. Inherited cataracts are often autosomal dominant and usually bilateral. The family history may however not be apparent as the parents may be unaware that they themselves have cataracts. Bilateral cataracts are more commonly associated with systemic disease and should therefore prompt a diagnostic investigations and examination of the parents for undetected cataracts. Unilateral cataracts are usually sporadic and are not frequently associated with any systemic diseases or other anomalies.

- **Vitreous** - Persistence of the fetal vasculature can cause an opaque membrane behind the lens. This occurs when there is a failure of the fetal vasculature to regress at birth.

- **Retinal** – Retinoblastoma is the most worrying cause of an absent red reflex. The inherited form is autosomal dominant and presents bilaterally in the first year of life. Sporadic cases are usually unilateral and present between the ages of 1 and 3 years. Large, unilateral tumours are treated with enucleation whereas smaller tumours can be treated locally using photocoagulation, thermotherapy, or plaque therapy. Other causes of a pale retina include retinopathy of prematurity and retinal detachment as in this case.

The newborn baby Jaxon has unilateral leukocoria making it unlikely that there is an underlying systemic disorder causing the eye disorder. He is well grown and otherwise well, except for a soft systolic murmur which does not sound as if it would relate to an underlying cardiac defect that one may see in congenital rubella or fetal alcohol syndrome. Mum did drink during the pregnancy but not at levels that one would normally expect to result in fetal alcohol syndrome and there are no other features to suggest this or congenital rubella syndrome. The cataracts in galactosemia or retinoblastoma would also not be present at delivery.

Syllabus Mapping

Ophthalmology

- Know the presenting features of visual impairment and the principles of management

- Know the common causes of an absent red reflex, be able to refer appropriately and be aware of management options

- Know the common causes of ptosis and proptosis and the principles of management

- Know the causes and presentations of strabismus and the principles of management

References and Further Reading

1. Long V. The Eye and Vision. In: Levene M, Hall D, (eds.) MRCPCH Mastercourse Volume 2. Churchill Livingstone, London. 2007 p 60 54-61

2. http://www.aao.org/eye-health/ask-ophthalmologist-q/why-white-reflex-seen-in-photo-not-during-exam. Accessed 28th October 2016

3. Tuli SY, Giordano BP, Kelly M, Fillipps D, Tuli SS. Newborn with an absent red reflex. Journal of pediatric health care: official publication of National Association of Pediatric Nurse Associates & Practitioners. 2013 Jan;27(1):51

Chapter 45: Boisterous Ben
Dr Robert Dinwiddie and
Dr Justine Clair-Southin

45

You are seeing patients in the general paediatric clinic. The GP has referred Ben, a 6 year old boy with behaviour problems. In the last 6 months he has become irritable, argumentative and he has smashed doors and other household items. He likes playing football and has long sessions playing his game's console.

His grandfather, to whom he was very close, died 1 year ago and his parents recently separated. He sees his father once a month. Although he was doing well in school his work and sports activities have recently declined and he has also become disruptive in class.

Q1. Which one of the following is the most likely diagnosis?

A.   Acute anxiety state
B.   Attention deficit hyperactivity disorder (ADHD)
C.   Autism spectrum disorder
D.   Depression
E.   Oppositional defiant disorder (ODD)

Q2. Which one of the following is the most appropriate first intervention?

A.   Cognitive behavioural therapy for Ben
B.   Cognitive behavioural therapy for Ben's mother
C.   Parent training programme
D.   Prescribe methylphenidate
E.   Prescribe risperidone

Ben returns to the clinic 6 months later. His behaviour has deteriorated and he has been excluded from school. He has set fire to the local park benches and been in trouble with the police. His mother says that he "explodes" at home and has thrown his game controller at his 3 month old sister when she was crying. You refer him to the Child and Adolescent Mental Health Service (CAMHS).

Q3. Which one of the following CAMHS professionals is most appropriate for Ben to be seen by?

A.   Bereavement counsellor
B.   Play therapist
C.   Psychiatrist
D.   Psychologist
E.   Social Worker

Answers and Rationale

Q1.   **E: Oppositional defiant disorder (ODD)**
Q2.   **C: Parent training programme**
Q3.   **C: Psychiatrist**

Ben's behaviour is outside the norms for children of his age. Mental health problems presenting in the paediatric age group are more common than many people realise. At least 10% have a mental health problem at some time during childhood and adolescence (1, 2, 3); 30% of a typical GP's child consultations are for behavioural problems; 45% of community child health referrals are for behaviour disturbances; and psychiatric disorders are a factor in 28% of all paediatric outpatient referrals (4).

When assessing such disorders it is useful to perform what is called a "diagnostic formulation" (1). This utilises a method called the "four Ps" to delineate possible contributing factors to the illness. These are described as;

* **p**redisposing
* **p**recipitating
* **p**erpetuating
* **p**rotective.

Examples of predisposing factors include chronic illness, physical, sexual, or emotional abuse, single parent upbringing, and socio-economic deprivation. Precipitating/trigger factors include acute illness, bereavement, and parental discord with or without separation; also bullying, including being "picked on" at school. Perpetuating factors include unsympathetic attitudes and lack of support from parents, family and other caregivers. Protective factors include a calm temperament, self-confidence, good parenting, and support from other caregivers (1, 2).

Ben is most likely to be suffering from oppositional defiant disorder (ODD). This disorder is characterised by episodes of anger, aggressiveness, and spiteful behaviour towards others. Symptoms often start around the age of 5 or 6 and it is thought to be more common in boys than girls. The condition is especially likely if symptoms persist for more than 6 months. Predisposing factors include lack of family support and discipline, marital conflict and parental disinterest or rejection. Precipitating factors include the loss of a family member to whom the patient was particularly close. Other adverse influences may be due to learning difficulties and lack of interaction with peers at school. A significant proportion of affected children and young people with ODD will go on to have personality problems in adult life (4).

The management of children with long-term mental health problems can be complex and difficult thus requiring a multidisciplinary approach. The Child and Adolescent Mental Health Service (CAMHS) provides all necessary services that work with children and young people who have difficulties with emotional or behavioural wellbeing. This work often includes working with both the child and their family. The multidisciplinary CAMHS team consists of psychiatrists, psychologists, social workers, nurses, support workers, occupational therapists, psychological therapists, mental health workers and substance misuse workers.

The initial management of conduct disorders consists of parent and family training programmes, with cognitive behavioural therapy of use in older children (9-14 years). When Ben returns to the clinic he has not responded to the interventions put in place and he is now demonstrating severe aggressive behaviour. Medication has little place for the routine management of behavioural problems in children and young people with conduct disorders. However, in cases like Ben where there is severe aggression and failure to respond to psychological interventions, risperidone may be considered for the short-term management of these symptoms. This should only be prescribed by a clinician with expertise in conduct disorders, following a comprehensive assessment and diagnosis. The effects of risperidone should be reviewed after 3-4 weeks, and discontinued if there is no indication of a clinically important response at six weeks (4).

Anxiety disorders are amongst the most common mental health disorders, occurring in 5% to 19% of all children and adolescents. In children younger than 12 separation anxiety is the most common disorder. An acute anxiety state can arise due to fear of illness, bereavement and fear of losing control of one's life. Potential factors in this case include the loss of a close relative and the marital break-up. Somatic symptoms include restlessness, fatigue, headaches, and abdominal pain. Irritability, anger, and oppositional behaviour can be an expression of an anxiety disorder, but is much less common (1). Fluoxetine, although primarily used for the treatment of depression, is sometimes prescribed for acute anxiety but not for other disorders such as ODD (5).

Three key features define attention-deficit hyperactivity disorder (ADHD): inattention, hyperactivity, and impulsivity. Inattention is evident as a short attention span, continuously switching from one activity to another, and difficulty in following instructions. Hyperactivity is manifest as a child "always on the go", who "cannot sit still" even in the classroom, and excessive talking. Impulsivity in the child is demonstrated as interruption of others and not waiting for their turn in games (1). Defiant and aggressive behaviour can be an associated but is not a primary feature of this disorder. Ben's symptoms of aggression and the fact that he can sit and play his games console for long periods of time make ADHD unlikely.

The management of ADHD is primarily with psychological, behavioural, and educational support. Pharmacotherapy, which includes the use of methylphenidate, dexamfetamine, or atomoxetine, is also useful in this condition. An exclusion diet has been found to be useful on some occasions, especially in preschool children, where one or two factors such as specific foods or a food additive appear to trigger an abnormal behavioural response (8).

Autism spectrum disorder (ASD) is the name for a group of developmental disorders. ASD includes a wide range, a spectrum, of symptoms, skills, and levels of disability.

Classical features include impaired social interaction, particularly lack of interest in other people, a tendency to play alone and an appearance of "living in their own world". Other features include speech delay, learning difficulties, and repetitive rituals. Aggressiveness does not tend to be a feature (1, 2). A careful developmental history is necessary in making a diagnosis.

The prevalence of childhood depression has been estimated to be approximately 1% in pre-pubertal children and 3% in adolescents. It is experienced by twice as many adolescent girls than boys. Depression is characterised by persistent low mood, loss of interest or loss of pleasure, and fatigue or low energy. In childhood, depression can have a more insidious onset than in adults, and is characterised by irritability more than sadness, and often occurs with other behavioural disorders (6). In this case, the boy did experience agitation, poor concentration and deterioration of school work. However, depression also frequently results in social withdrawal, tiredness, fatigue, and excessive sleep, features not present in this case. A child or young person with depression should be reviewed by CAMHS, and offered psychological interventions, such as individual individual, Cognitive Behavioural Therapy (CBT), interpersonal therapy, family therapy, or psychotherapy, for at least 3 months. If the child's depression does not respond, they should have a multidisciplinary team review, and offered alternative or additional psychological treatment to the child and family. Fluoxetine can be considered, with caution if the symptoms remain unresponsive (6).

Syllabus Mapping

Behavioural Medicine/Psychiatry

- Know the determinants of child and adolescent mental health

- Understand how common emotional and behaviour problems may evolve

- Know the role of child and Adolescent Mental Health Services CAMHS

- Understand the principles of managing common emotional and behaviour problems such as temper tantrums, breath holding attack, the crying baby, oppositional behaviour, enuresis, and encopresis, excessive water drinking, school refusal, bullying and chronic fatigue syndrome and when to refer

- Know about the signs and symptoms of Attention Deficit Hyperactivity Disorder (ADHD) and appropriate referral pathways

- Know the features of depression in children and adolescents and when to refer to specialist services

References and Further Reading

1. Lewin C. Mental health. In Training in Paediatrics. Eds Gardiner M, Eisen S, Murphy C. Oxford University Press, Oxford 2009;ch19:407-424

2. Davie M, Stedmon J. Child and adolescent mental health. In The Science of Paediatrics. Eds Lissauer T, Carroll W. Elsevier, London 2016;ch24:463-478

3. Hoare P. Psychiatric disorders in childhood. In Forfar & Arneil's Textbook of Pediatrics, 7th edn. Eds McIntosh N, Helms P, Smyth R, Logan S. Churchill Livingstone Elsevier, Edinburgh 2008;ch34:1541-1568

4. National Institute for Clinical Excellence. Antisocial behaviour and conduct disorders in children and young people: recognition, intervention and management. NICE Clinical Guideline 158. 2013

5. James AC, James G, Cowdrey FA, Soler A, Choke A. Cognitive behavioural therapy for anxiety disorders in children and adolescents. Cochrane Database Syst Rev. 2013 Jan 1;6

6. National Institute for Clinical Excellence. Depression in children. NICE Clinical Guideline 28. 2015

Chapter 46: Melena Monday
Dr Rebecca Kettle

You are the gastroenterology ST2 doctor working in the local children's hospital. The emergency department refer the following children to you on Monday morning.

The following are a list of investigations:

A.   Abdominal ultrasound scan
B.   Abdominal x-ray
C.   CT abdomen
D.   Endoscopy
E.   Lower GI contrast

F.   No investigation required
G.   Skeletal survey
H.   Stool culture
I.   Technetium scan
J.   Upper GI contrast

Which is the most appropriate diagnostic investigation?

Q1a. A 16 month old girl presents with a history of melena for the last few days. Her mother says she seems to have had tummy pain in the morning but is better when she has eaten. She fractured her leg 2 weeks ago when she fell down the stairs and her leg remains in a plaster cast. She is otherwise usually well. Her mother has been giving her medicine to help with the pain.

Q1b. A 14 month old presents with a 10-hour history of screaming. She is now having non-bilious vomiting and has passed a red mucous stool. She is normally fit and well though had a cough and cold in the last week. On examination she is alert, pink and well perfused but lethargic. Her abdomen is soft and non-tender, with a mass in the right upper quadrant.

Q1c. A 15 month old boy presents after his father found his nappy full of bright red blood, his father says he has been well, playing normally all day and has no past medical history of note. On assessment he is pale, his capillary refill time is 4/seconds, heart rate 180/minute, respiratory rate 40/minute, oxygen saturations 94% in air, blood pressure 70/45 mmHg, chest is clear, heart sounds normal, pulses weak, abdomen is soft and non-tender with no palpable masses.

A 2 month old breast fed boy presents with a long history of crying after feeds, being generally unsettled and with loose stools, which have been bloody on several occasions. He was born at 39+5 weeks following a normal pregnancy, weighing was 3.4 kg (25th – 50th centile). He has been breastfed from birth and been prescribed sodium alginate by his GP for reflux disease. He has regular emollients for eczema.

On examination he weighs 6.6 kg (9th-25th centile) and is alert and responsive. He is unsettled and crying when you examine him. His heart rate is 130/minute, central capillary refill time 2/seconds and apart from some moderate eczema his systemic examination is otherwise well.

Q2. What is the most appropriate first line investigation?

A.   Lower GI endoscopy
B.   Trial of hypoallergenic infant formula milk
C.   Trial of maternal dairy free diet
D.   Trial of ranitidine
E.   Ultrasound scan of his abdomen

Answers and Rationale

Q1a   D: Endoscopy
Q1b   A: Abdominal ultrasound scan
Q1c   I: Technitium Scan
Q2.   C: Trial of maternal dairy free diet

This question requires a knowledge of the causes of gastrointestinal bleeding in children, which presents in variety of ways with varying causes. The importance of diagnosing the cause in a timely manner ensures appropriate management and prevents unnecessary investigations for the child, particularly if those investigations are likely to cause distress or expose the child to radiation.

When approaching a problem of gastrointestinal tract bleeding there are some questions you could consider when evaluating the likely cause. Firstly, is it blood? Certain food stuffs (e.g. beetroot) can cause vomit and stool to look altered in colour and may not anything to worry about. Secondly, is it coming from the GI tract – blood in the nappy of a small child could originate from the genital-urinary tracts for example. Thirdly, how much blood is there and where is it coming from? Bright red blood, coffee ground vomit and melena suggest bleeding proximal to the ligament of Treitz at the duodenojejunal flexure; melena would suggest significant blood loss of over 2%. Bright red blood or dark red blood mixed with stool would suggest bleeding is originating from either the ileum or colon. If the blood is bright red and not mixed with stool it is more likely due to an ano-rectal source (1).

The first question suggests an upper GI bleed with a history of melena (blood which has been altered after passage through the gastrointestinal tract). The other salient points to identify in the history are the abdominal pain, seemingly worse in the morning, relieved by eating and the history of her mother giving her 'medicine' for her leg fracture. At 16 months old the child is likely to mobile and a fracture from an accident is feasible, though a thorough history needs to always be taken to determine the nature of any accident. The relevance of the fracture history is that her mother has been giving 'medicine' for the pain; this is likely to be a combination of paracetamol and ibuprofen, although you would always clarify this on taking a full detailed history. Ibuprofen is an NSAID which if used regularly for any length of time can cause gastric ulcers. NSAIDs are COX inhibitors, COX-2 inhibition produces the desired effect as an anti-inflammatory, however as NSAIDs are often non-specific they also inhibit COX-1 which is important in protecting the gastric mucosa from gastric acid, and can therefore cause ulceration. Ulcers can be painful and bleed, the blood then passes through the GI tract and is seen as melena when opening bowels. Ulcer pain is often worse when the stomach is empty and is relieved by eating as described in the question stem. Investigation of choice for a gastric ulcer is endoscopy to directly look at the lining of the stomach and diagnose the ulcer (2).

In question 1b, the important point to detect in the history is the intermittent nature of the pain in association with a red mucous stool, sometimes described as a 'redcurrant jelly stool'. If the child is not in pain during your assessment you may well have a negative examination with obvious cause, however as in this case there is a mass in the right upper quadrant. All of this information should lead you to think about intussusception, when the bowel invaginates on itself like a telescope taking its blood supply with it, if not treated intussusception can lead to bowel necrosis and perforation. Initial investigation with an abdominal ultrasound scan, proceeding to an air enema if the USS is confirmatory to treat the intussusception is standard in the UK. Classically an abdominal scan would show a target appearance of the bowel. If an air enema is not successful, referral to paediatric surgeons for a laparotomy is indicated. An abdominal x-ray could be performed and may show signs of bowel obstruction but would not be diagnostic. Digital rectal examination in children is very rarely, if ever indicated and should not be done.

The third case (1c) has 2 key points; firstly a large unprovoked rectal bleed and secondly, the child is in shock. Whilst the immediate thoughts are to resuscitate the child you still need to identify the cause of the bleeding to ensure appropriate management. A large painless per rectum bleed in a child should make you consider Meckel's diverticulum. Meckel's diverticulum is a congenital condition which is due to the incomplete degeneration of either a vitelline duct or an omphalomesenteric duct; this should normally happen at around 5-7 weeks gestation. The diverticulum that is left behind often contains gastric, intestinal or occasionally pancreatic tissue. Whilst you may initially think that the bleeding from a Meckel's diverticulum would present with melena, bright fresh blood can be seen if there is a large volume bleed from the upper GI region, which occurs in about 10% of cases (1). The Technetium scan is an isotope scan which identifies the ectopic gastric tissue diagnosing Meckel's Diverticulum. Meckel's diverticulum can also present in different ways being a focus for obstruction, volvulus and intussusception.

The other investigations listed above all have their place within investigating GI bleeding in children, some of the specific scenarios you might consider them in would be for example an abdominal x-ray can be diagnostic in necrotising enterocolitis which might present as PR bleeding in a neonate with abdominal distension and bilious aspirates, you can see evidence of perforation, pneumatosis and thickened bowel wall. An abdominal CT might indicated for cases inflammatory bowel disease which may present with lower GI bleeding. Upper GI contrast studies are used if malrotation, possible hiatus hernia. Lower GI contrast may be used to evaluate inflammatory bowel disease, lower GI bleeding where polyps may be suspected and can also be used to investigate for hirschprungs disease. A history of bloody diarrhoea with associated renal impairment would suggest haemolytic uraemic syndrome, in which case you would be looking to identify E Coli 0157 as causative pathogen on stool culture. A skeletal survey would be considered if you had concerns over non-accidental injury causing bleeding.

The history in question 2 is intended to lead you towards cow's milk protein allergy diagnosis. The points to note in include the history of gastro-oesophageal reflux, treatment for eczema (especially if it is refractory to standard treatment), the new onset of bloody stools and also that the infant is never settled after feeds. Cow's milk protein allergy (CMPA) is an immune mediated allergic response and can be either IgE mediated or non-IgE mediated. IgE mediated is related to histamine release with an acute and rapid onset of symptoms, non-IgE are non-acute with a delay in onset of 48 hours to 1 week post-ingestion. This question highlights one of the risk factors for CMPA – a history of atopic co-morbidities, in this case eczema but asthma is also risk factor along with a family history of atopy. Presentation of CMPA can vary but generally involves skin, gastrointestinal and respiratory system symptoms, if CMPA is suspected a focused allergy history should be taken. Diagnosis should be made according to the type of CMPA suspected, if IgE mediated allergy is suspected a skin prick test is indicated, if non-IgE mediated is suspected then a cows milk elimination diet for 2-6 weeks can be diagnostic, either for the child or if being breast-fed the mother should eliminate cows milk from her diet. Strict elimination from the child's diet (or maternal diet in exclusively breast fed babies) is the safest management of CMPA. Non-IgE CMPA can be managed within primary care with dietetic input, however IgE-mediated should be referred to secondary care. Secondary care referral is indicated for either CMPA if there is (3):

- Faltering growth with one or more GI symptoms
- One or more systemic reations
- One or more severe delayed reactions
- Significant atopic eczema with suspicion of multiple or cross-reactive food allergies
- Persistent parental concerns – even if the history is not supported
- Suspicion of multiple food allergies

Syllabus mapping

Gastroenterology and Hepatology

- Know the causes of acute abdominal pain and recognise when to refer, including urgency of referral

- Know the common causes of food allergies and intoelrances, their intial management and when to appropriately refer

- Know the common causes of upper and lower gastrointestinal bleeding, initial management and appropriate referral

References and Further Reading

1. Arain Z, Rossi TM. Gastrointestinal Bleeding in Children: An Overview of Condition Requiring Nonoperative Management. InSeminars in pediatric surgery 1999 Nov 30 (Vol. 8, No. 4, pp. 172-180). WB Saunders

2. Sullivan PB. Peptic ulcer disease in children. Paediatrics and Child Health. 2010 Oct 31;20(10):462-4

3. NICE Clinical Knowledge summary; Cows' milk protein allergy in children. June 2015. Accessed 10th November 2016 at https://cks.nice.org.uk/cows-milk-protein-allergy-in-children

Chapter 47: "Will you scan my daughter?"
Dr Emily Hoyle and Dr Prab Prabhakar

Laura is a 14 year old girl who attends her GP along with her mother. She has a 1-year history of intermittent headaches. She describes a tightening pain on both sides of her head that she scores as being 4/10. (0-no pain and 10 worst pains ever). The pain occurred approximately once a week but in the past month has occurred more frequently. She has not vomited with the headache and there are no visual disturbances. The headache is promptly relieved by paracetamol and ibuprofen.

Her height and weight are on the 98th centile and her neurological examination is entirely normal.

Q1. Which one of the following is the most likely diagnosis?

A.   Intracranial tumour
B.   Idiopathic intracranial hypertension
C.   Medication overuse headache
D.   Migraine
E.   Tension type headache

She returns 3 months later with almost a daily headaches (4/10 in intensity) which are not responding to paracetamol and Ibuprofen. Examination again is normal. Her mother is requesting a brain scan.

Q2. Which one of the following is the most likely diagnosis?

A.   Intracranial tumour
B.   Idiopathic intracranial hypertension
C.   Medication overuse headache
D.   Migraine
E.   Tension type headache

After 6 weeks of appropriate treatment, Laura's headache is back to her base line. She returns however 8 months later to the GP. The GP refers her to the rapid access paediatric clinic with the following letter:

"Thank you for seeing Laura who has had intermittent headaches for the past 2 years. However, over the past weeks the headaches been more persistent and worse in the mornings. The headaches are not relieved by her usual medication. There has also been associated early morning vomiting and visual disturbances".

Her neurological examination is normal but on fundoscopy she has bilateral papilloedema. Her mother wants you to arrange a brain scan.

Q4. Which one of the following is the most important initial investigation?

A.   CT scan and venography
B.   Headache diary
C.   Lumbar puncture with CSF manometry
D.   MRI and venography
E.   Trial of stopping analgesic medication

Answers and Rationale

Q1. **E: Tension type headache**
Q2. **C: Medication Overuse headache**
Q3. **D: MRI and venography**

Headache is a common problem faced in both the paediatric clinic and in the emergency department. Epidemiological studies show that 70% of school children have headaches at least once a year. Pre-pubertal boys are more affected than girls, but after puberty, headaches are more common in girls (1). An understanding of the different ways headaches can present in the different age groups is required to successfully managing these children.

History, as always, gives the diagnosis in the majority of situations with investigations required to" rule out" or "rule in" important secondary headaches.

It is an important first step to establish from the history and examination whether there are any "red flag" symptoms or signs present. (Box 47.1). This will always prompt further investigation, usually with cross sectional brain imaging as the first line investigation (1,2).

Symptoms	Signs
• Short history or recurrent severe headache for few weeks • Symptoms of raised intracranial pressure (early morning headache , morning vomiting, headache worse with cough or Valsalva) • Personality or behaviour change, • Weakness, visual disturbances, seizures • Underlying history of neurocutaneous syndrome • Associated systemic illness • < 3 years age	• Papilloedema • VI nerve palsy • Decreased conscious level • Deteriorating condition • Associated neurological signs

Box 47.1 "Red Flag" Symptoms and signs in Childhood headache

Within the history, it is important to ask location, duration of headaches, severity and intensity. For example, a chronic, recurring headache, which is shortlasting (<30 minutes) with mild intensity, and without any associated neurological abnormalities is likely to be benign in nature. However occipital headaches are very rare in children and although can be a feature of tension headache, it should raise the suspicion of a posterior fossa tumour (1). A pain-scoring system should be adopted when performing a history. Other questions important in a history are necessity for medication, triggers, relieving factors and questions relating to school, friends and stressful situations.

It is important to perform a full physical examination. Neurological examination if performed correctly has a high sensitivity for intracranial pathology. Blood pressure (using age appropriate cuff) measurements, head circumference measurements in the younger child (<2 years) and systemic examination for neurocutaneous syndrome should also be performed. Ensure you check the fundi for evidence of raised intracranial pressure manifested by papilledema and in a child whose headache pattern suggests a frontal location and/or in the eyes, an ophthalmology examination should be performed to assess for refractive errors.

In the absence of red flag signs, the history and examination should be directed at identifying if the headache is likely to be primary or secondary. In a child with primary headaches, the physical examination is normal and there is no "cause" for the headache identified. Further investigation is seldom necessary. In secondary headache, the headache is attributable to another cause and clinical examination and investigations can be abnormal.

Laura originally presents with a history and examination that lacks any "red flag" signs or symptoms. This is indicative of a primary headache. Causes of primary headaches include migraine, tension type headache, new onset daily persistent headache and trigeminal autonomic cephalagias (cluster headache or paroxysmal hemicrania).

Tension type headache is characterised by mild (no interference with normal activities) to moderate (interferes with some but not all activities) intensity of headache. The pain is dull or pressure around the head and is not associated with other symptoms such as nausea, vomiting or intolerance to light and noise. This is the most likely diagnosis when Sally originally presents.

Migraine is another consideration but Sally's history does not suggest this as the underlying diagnosis. The headache often builds up in severity over 30-60 minutes reaching maximum intensity within 1-2 hours. The pain is described as severe (stops all activities) or moderate (stops some but not all activities) and throbbing in quality, but many children find it difficult describe pain. The site of maximum pain is often on the forehead unlike the unilateral headache in adult patients. During attacks, the child is pale, loses appetite, feels nauseated, may vomit and complains of intolerance to light, noise and exercise. They may feel better after rest or sleep and return to their normal self between attacks. Aura symptoms (commonly visual and less often sensory or motor) precedes headache in around 15-20% of patients. Migraine with typical visual aura is easily distinguishable and relatively common, but in some children atypical aura and specific syndromes can pose difficulties in diagnosis and treatment. In fact, around 80% of children with migraine have migraine without aura (3). There are no clear triggers of migraine attacks in the majority of children, but around one third of patients may report stress, missing a meals or lack of sleep.

Cluster headaches are a rare but very severe type of headache which is always unilateral on or around an eye, lasting 15-180 minutes and is associated with autonomic features on the same side of the pain. The natural course of cluster headache is characterised by spells of severe and very frequent attacks of headache lasting for 1-2 weeks and recurring every 1-2 months. Treatment includes breathing in pure oxygen at a rate of between 7 to 15 litres per minute. The most successful abortive treatment of a cluster attack is a self-administered subcutaneous injection of sumatriptan.

Paroxysmal hemicrania is another rare headache which is unilateral and usually all over the head associated with ipsilateral autonomic features (ptosis, miosis, eye watering, eye redness, nose watering, eye lid oedoma, ear full ness). This headache responds readily to indomethacin.

New Onset Daily Persistent Headache (NDPH) is a persistent headache, daily from its onset which is clearly remembered. The pain lacks characteristic features, and may be migraine-like or tension-type-like, or have elements of both. NDPH is unique in that headache is daily from onset, and very soon unremitting, typically occurring in individuals without a prior headache history.

When Sally re-attends 3 months later, there is a change in the frequency of the headache but not the quality or intensity of the headache. Most importantly, the analgesics are now ineffective. There are no clinical signs indicative of a secondary headache. In this scenario, medication overuse will have to be considered.

Medication Overuse Headache (MOH) occurs on 15 or more days per month developing as a consequence of regular overuse (more than 2-3 days per week not the number of doses(4)) of acute or symptomatic headache medication for more than three months. It usually, but not invariably, resolves after the overuse is stopped. Medication overuse headache can occur with paracetamol, aspirin, triptan and NSAIDs. Opioids are not recommended for use in primary headache disorders due to the high incidence of MOH and tolerance.

When Laura returns 6 months later there are red flag features suggesting a secondary headache, namely the early morning headache with vomiting and papilledema, both of which point towards there being raised intracranial pressure. Raised intracranial pressure is most likely caused by either a intracranial mass of idiopathic intracranial hypertension (IIH). The absence of neurological signs and associated symptoms makes IIH more likely than an intracranial mass.

Idiopathic intracranial hypertension (IIH) is defined as an elevated intracranial pressure (> 25cm water in normal and >28 cm water in obese children(5)) without clinical, radiologic or laboratory evidence of a secondary cause. It can occur in all age groups, both genders and in both obese and non-obese individuals. It is rare in children < 10 years of age and extremely rare in those <3 years (1,5). Headache is the commonest symptom described by children with this condition though they can also present with neck, shoulder, or arm pain; nausea, vomiting, tinnitus, diplopia, blurred vision, and transient vision abnormalities. Occasionally, children will present following a routine optometry assessment that identifies papilloedema. A thorough history and examination is important in these patients to identify potential secondary causes of raised intracranial pressure. If IIH is suspected a MRI with venography should be performed to exclude the presence of intracranial masses or intracranial venous thrombosis. In cases where visual loss is a concern, emergency neurosurgical CSF diversion may be required (1). Acetazolamide and Topiramate are now used as first line management with weight loss advised in those who are overweight.

Syllabus Mapping

Neurology

- Know the causes of headache and be able to treat or refer as necessary

Emergency Medicine

- Know how to recognise and initiate treatment for children presenting with neurological emergencies

References

1. Lewis DW, Rothner AD. Headache in children and adolescents. Current Therapy in Neurological Disease, Vol 6. Edited by Johnson RT, Griffin JW, McArthur JC. Mosby, Inc. pages 88-94.

2. Chong Shang Chee. Headaches in children: A Clinical Approach. The International Classification of Headache Disorders, 2nd Edition. Cephalalgia 2004, 24(1): 1-160

3. Lewis DW. Pediatric migraine. Neurologic clinics. 2009 May 31;27(2):481-501

4. Diener HC, Holle D, Solbach K, Gaul C. Medication-overuse headache: risk factors, pathophysiology and management. Nature Reviews Neurology. 2016 Oct 1;12(10):575-83

5. Babiker MO, Prasad M, MacLeod S, Chow G, Whitehouse WP. Fifteen-minute consultation: the child with idiopathic intracranial hypertension. Archives of disease in childhood-Education & practice edition. 2014 Mar 25:edpract-2013

Further Reading

Headache Classification Committee of the International Headache Society (2013), The International Classification of Headache Disorders, 3rd edition (beta version)

Hershey A, Powers S, Winner P. Pediatric Headaches in Clinical Practice. Wiley Blackwell. March 2009

Chapter 48: Alarming allergies
Dr Jim Gould

48

Saanvi is a 13 month old girl who attends the emergency department with her parents. One hour ago she ate 4 spoonfuls of scrambled egg and 25 minutes later she developed a widespread urticarial rash over her face and trunk. She had no previous history of reaction to egg, although her mother could not recall giving her egg on its own in the past. She had a past history of generalised infantile eczema, which had developed over the last 3-4 months and was being treated with emollients

On examination her breathing pattern was normal and her chest was clear on auscultation. Her eczema is generalised and severe with no unaffected areas of skin on her trunk or limbs.

Q1. Which one other clinical feature, if it had occurred, would have met the criteria for anaphylactic reaction to the egg?

A.   Extreme pallor
B.   Vomiting
C.   Pruritus
D.   Swollen Lips
E.   Hypertension

Q2. What would be the most appropriate specific egg allergy test to confirm egg allergy?

A.   IgG blood testing for egg
B.   IgE blood testing for egg
C.   Oral challenge test for egg
D.   Patch test for egg
E.   Skin prick test for egg

Q3. What is the most important management plan for Sannvi on discharge?

A.   Dietary avoidance of all dairy and egg containing foods
B.   Dietary avoidance of all egg containing foods
C.   Prescribe an adrenaline (Epinephrine) injector pen (150mcg)
D.   Prescribe oral antihistamine
E.   Prescribe topical steroid cream

Q4. If Saanvi goes on to develop further food allergies in the future, which is she least likely to outgrow?

A.   Cow's milk
B.   Egg
C.   Peanut
D.   Wheat
E.   Soya

Answers and Rationale

Q1.   A: Extreme pallor
Q2.   B: IgE blood testing for egg
Q3.   B: Dietary avoidance of all egg containing foods
Q4.   C: Peanut

Allergy can present in many different, and sometimes confusing, ways. It can affect most systems, including upper airway (allergic rhinitis, laryngeal oedema), lower respiratory tract (asthma), gastrointestinal system (vomiting, enteropathies, colitis), skin (various rashes, eczema) and systemic/cardiovascular (anaphylaxis, etc.).

The immune mechanisms leading to hypersensitivity were classified by Gell and Coombs in 1963, and this classification in modified form continues to this day (Table 48.1). Most common allergic conditions seen in children where there is a response to an external antigen (e.g. food protein, pollen) are IgE mediated Type I reactions, with some food allergies producing enteropathy or colitis being non-IgE mediated (type III or IV, or possible a mixture of type I and III or IV).

Type	Mechanism	Examples
I	IgE	Anaphylaxis, asthma, hay fever, eczema, some food allergies
II	Cytotoxic, antibody dependant	Autoimmune haemolytic anaemia, Goodpasture's syndrome, rheumatic heart disease
III	Immune complexes	Lupus, serum sickness, post strep. glomerulonephritis
IV	Cell mediated	Contact dermatitis, Mantoux test, some intestinal food allergy
V*	Receptor mediated autoimmune disease	Graves' disease, myasthenia gravis

Table 48.1: Gell and Coombs classification of hypersensitivity

*Type V is an additional classification recently added to distinguish these diseases previously categorised as type II.

Food allergy is a clinically important topic for a paediatrician. Reactions to food substances are quite common, and not all relate to allergy, which is an adverse reaction that involves the immune system. The term intolerance is preferred when an adverse reaction shows no evidence of immune system involvement. Examples of intolerance include lactose intolerance (related to a primary or secondary deficiency of intestinal lactase) which produces bloating and loose explosive stools in infants and children.

Pharmacological food intolerance can also be seen - examples include tyramine in strong cheese and caffeine in coffee, both of which can induce adverse reactions in children (1).

Common allergies include milk, eggs, peanut, soy, wheat, tree nuts (such as walnuts and cashews), fish and shellfish. The example used in this above is an infant with egg allergy though a similar presentation could occur with any of these food types. Infants with cow's milk protein allergy can sometimes present, especially in early infancy, with a haemorrhagic colitis (non IgE mediated reaction), either because the infant is formula fed, or more rarely breast fed by a mother consuming cow's milk in her diet (human milk can contain cow's milk protein). Allergy such as this can be more difficult to diagnose, as skin testing or specific IgE analysis may be negative or equivocal, so that diagnosis will rest on history and dietary trials.

Anaphylaxis is a severe, life-threatening, generalised hypersensitivity reaction, characterised by rapidly developing, life-threatening problems involving: the airway, breathing and/or circulation. In most cases, there are associated skin and mucosal changes (2). The criteria for diagnosing an anaphylactic reaction are outlined in (Table 48.2).

Anaphylaxis is highly likely when any 1 of the following 3 criteria is fulfilled following exposure to an allergen:
1. Acute onset of an illness (minutes to several hours) with involvement of the skin, mucosal tissue, or both (e.g., generalised hives, pruritus or flushing, swollen lips-tongue-uvula) and at least 1 of the following: a. Respiratory compromise (e.g. dyspnoea, wheeze, bronchospasm, stridor, reduced PEF, hypoxemia) b. Reduced BP or associated symptoms of end-organ dysfunction (e.g. hypotonia [collapse], syncope, incontinence)
2. 2 or more of the following that occur rapidly after exposure to a *likely* **allergen for that patient (minutes to several hours):** a. Involvement of the skin-mucosal tissue (e.g., generalised hives, itch-flush, swollen lips-tongue-uvula) b. Respiratory compromise (e.g., dyspnea, wheeze, bronchospasm, stridor, reduced PEF, hypoxemia) c. Reduced BP or associated symptoms (e.g., hypotonia [collapse], syncope, incontinence) d. Persistent GI symptoms (e.g., painful abdominal cramps, vomiting)
3. Reduced BP after exposure to a *known* allergen for that patient (minutes to several hours): a. Infants and children: low systolic BP (age specific) or > 30% decrease in systolic BP˙

Table 48.2: Clinical criteria for diagnosing anaphylaxis (3)

PEF = Peak expiratory flow; BP: blood pressure; GI: gastrointestinal* Low systolic blood pressure for children is age specific and defined as: < 70 mmHg for age 1 month to 1 year;
<70mmHg + [2 x age] for age 1 to 10 years < 90mmHg for age 11 to 17 years.
Adapted from Kim & Fischer, 2011

In the first question the pruritus and swollen lips are part of the skin/mucosal involvement whilst the vomiting is not described as being persistent. The extreme pallor signifies circulatory collapse and would indicate hypotension occurring as part of an anaphylactic response.

The most important and immediate intervention in this child needs to be dietary intervention, with immediate removal of all foods containing even traces of egg from the diet, under the supervision of a paediatric dietician. Allergy testing may show up other possible food allergies, so that at a later date, other food substances may also need to be removed from the diet, but this should only be undertaken with paediatric dietetic intervention and advice, and only if there is not substantial clinical improvement of the infant's eczema with removal of egg from the diet. Complete removal of egg should only be for a specific period (perhaps until the child's second birthday) when attempts should be made to induce tolerance to egg by gradual re-introduction of egg back into the diet, starting with traces of egg in cooked food products. Other interventions including antihistamines and topical steroids may well be necessary if the child's eczema remains very troublesome, but should not be introduced immediately whilst awaiting any possible response of the eczema to the initial dietary intervention. It is common to find cow's milk allergy along with egg allergy. However an egg free diet combined with a cow's milk protein free diet is complex and difficult to initiate, and would only be done if allergy testing suggested significant milk allergy, and response to an egg free diet was disappointing. It is also clearly possible that further accidental egg administration in this infant could induce anaphylaxis. There may therefore be a need for an adrenaline (epinephrine) pen prescription at some point in the near future, but in a 13 month old child, an egg free diet should be possible to maintain with the supervision and understanding of carers, and there should be no need for prescription of a pen as part of immediate therapeutic intervention.

When investigating food allergies, skin prick testing will give more directly relevant information about the degree of sensitivity of the child to a particular allergen than specific blood IgE testing (previously termed RAST IgE or immunoCAP). Specific blood IgE measurements, although predictive of allergy (4), can give an elevated result without the patient having any symptoms, and the level of specific IgE to that allergen has little bearing on the clinical level of sensitivity or the likelihood of future anaphylaxis. The size of a skin prick wheal when testing may have some relationship to the degree of allergy (although this is controversial). The problem with skin prick testing is that it requires an area of skin relatively unaffected by eczema, and occasionally therefore cannot be undertaken if there is generalised florid eczema, nor can it be undertaken if the infant has recently been given antihistamines. IgG blood testing for egg has no proven value, and should not be undertaken. Patch testing is reserved for testing for contact dermatitis, and would rarely be undertaken in infants (5). An oral challenge test (undertaken in a controlled hospital environment) could potentially be dangerous, and with this history is not indicated unless all allergy tests subsequently proved negative.

Tolerance to many foods tends to improve with age in food allergic children, the exceptions being peanut and crustacean/shellfish. In one review paper, 80% of children who had been cow's milk intolerant developed tolerance by 5 years, with egg it was 66% by age 7 years, soya, 69% by 10 years and wheat 65% by 12 years (6). With peanut and shellfish, the spontaneous development of tolerance appears to be much less common (7). With peanut, tolerance can often be successfully achieved by active oral de-sensitisation, but once achieved, this needs to be maintained in most children with regular oral consumption of peanut (8).

Syllabus Mapping

Gastroenterology and Hepatology (including surgical abdominal conditions)

*   Know the common causes of food allergies and intolerances, their initial management and when to appropriately refer

Emergency Medicine

*   Know the causes and features of anaphylaxis and its management

Infection Immunology and Allergy

*   Know the common allergies and advise on management

References and Further Reading

1. Food intolerance. Allergy UK. https://www.allergyuk.org/intolerance-and-sensitivity-menu/intolerance-and-sensitivity. Last accessed November 29th 2016

2. Resuscitation Council (UK) 2008. Emergency treatment of anaphylactic reactions. Guidelines for healthcare providers

3. Kim H., Fischer D. Anaphylaxis. Allergy, Asthma and Clinical Immunology. 2011;7 (Suppl. 1):S6

4. Baral VR, Hourihane JO. Food allergy in children. Postgraduate medical journal. 2005 Nov 1;81(961):693-701

5. Patch testing. Allergy UK. https://www.allergyuk.org/diagnosis--testing-of-allergy/patch-testing. Last accessed November 29th 2016

6. Panel NS. Guidelines for the diagnosis and management of food allergy in the United States: report of the NIAID-sponsored expert panel. Journal of Allergy and Clinical Immunology. 2010 Dec 31;126(6):S1-58

7. Gupta RS, Lau CH, Sita EE, Smith B, Greenhawt MJ. Factors associated with reported food allergy tolerance among US children. Annals of Allergy, Asthma & Immunology. 2013 Sep 30;111(3):194-8

8. Anagnostou K, Islam S, King Y, Foley L, Pasea L, Palmer C, Bond S, Ewan P, Clark A. Study of induction of Tolerance to Oral Peanut: a randomised controlled trial of desensitisation using peanut oral immunotherapy in children (STOP II). National Institute for Health Research.2014;1,(4)

Chapter 49: A Baby with a rash
Dr Hugh Bishop

Ife is an 8 week old baby boy of African British ethnicity presents to the Assessment Unit after referral from the GP who saw him an hour before, with a history of irritability and poor feeding. His mother explains that his urine has been smelly for a day or so and he seems to be in pain, screaming when she tries to feed him. His length, weight and OFC are all on the 50th percentile on the WHO Growth Chart.

Examination reveals a fractious baby and a mixed petechial and purpuric rash on his trunk and limbs. There is no mucosal bleeding. Intravenous access is obtained and blood tests are sent. The following results are telephoned from the haematology laboratory:

Haemoglobin	87 g/l	PT	22 secs
MCV	83 fl	APPT	56 secs
White cell count	19 x 10⁹/l	Fibrinogen	0.5
Neutrophils	13 x 10⁹/l		
Platelets	32 x 10⁹/l		
Reticulocyte count	30		

Q1. What is the most likely diagnosis?

A.   Disseminated Intravascular Coagulation
B.   Galactosemia
C.   Haemophilia A
D.   Sickle Cell Disease
E.   von Willebrand Disease Type III

Q2. What is the likeliest cause of the haemoglobin result?

A.   G6PD Deficiency
B.   Iron deficiency anaemia
C.   Physiological anaemia
D.   Sickle Cell Disease
E.   Vitamin B12 deficiency

Q3. What is the most important initial treatment?

A.   Blood transfusion
B.   Fresh Frozen Plasma
C.   Intraenous Paracetamol
D.   Intravenous Cefotaxime
E.   Platelet transfusion

Answers and Rationale

Q1.   **A: Disseminated Intravascular Coagulation**
Q2.   **C: Physiological Anaemia**
Q3.   **D: Intravenous Cefotaxime**

In clinical practice, and in exams, the ethnicity of the patient can be highly relevant to the diagnosis, and therefore the treatment, of your patient. However, it can also be a confounder, with no relevance. You must always read questions carefully, look at the data presented, and then relate it to the specific question that is being asked.

In the first question, there is a clear blood picture of disseminated Intravascular coagulation (DIC), with thrombocytopaenia, prolonged prothrombin and activated partial thromboplastin times, and a low fibrinogen. It is possible that the patient could have Sickle Cell Disease, but a crisis at this age is extremely unlikely, due to the protective effect of raised levels of fetal haemoglobin in infancy. Haemophilia A would explain the prolonged APTT but would not account for all of the abnormalities seen. The learning point here is that Haemophilia A does not have a differential incidence related to ethnicity. Type III vWD can present with significant coagulopathy, but the thrombocytopenia is not typical of this variant, and the incidence of Type 3 vWD is around 1 in 50,0000. Galactosemia predisposes to E Coli sepsis, and is a potential diagnosis here, but as above, you must always look at the data. You have clear evidence that there is a diagnosis of DIC, whereas you would be postulating that there might be a diagnosis of Galactosemia.

Regarding the explanation of the haemoglobin result, it is important to revise normal haematopoiesis and how this changes through childhood. There is a physiological anaemia in infancy, with the haemoglobin reaching its nadir at 8-12 weeks of age, and the haemoglobin in this question is entirely normal for this age. As with everything in medicine, it is vital to understand what is normal prior to considering what is abnormal. Sickle Cell Disease could be present in this baby, but for the reasons outlined above, crises are uncommon at this age, and the haemoglobin would be significantly lower were this part of his presentation. Iron deficiency anaemia does occur in infants, with premature babies at particular risk, but the normal MCV is against this being likely, and there is nothing in the history to particularly point to iron deficiency. B12 deficiency is an important cause of anaemia to recognise, but it is characterised by a raised MCV, and is rare in infancy. G6PD deficiency is relatively common in those of African British ethnicity, but would be characterised by prolonged jaundice in conjunction with haemolytic anaemia, of which there is no evidence here.

In relation to treatment, you must always consider what will harm the patient in this moment, and what can be done immediately to mitigate that risk of harm. In the case of a clear picture of DIC, particularly with an irritable infant, the most likely underlying cause is septicaemia, which can be rapidly fatal. While the coagulopathy and thrombocytopenia may well require therapy with blood products, this will take time to arrange through the blood bank, and failing to treat the underlying sepsis rapidly, could prove fatal. The baby is irritable, and treating their discomfort is very important, but IV Paracetamol will not treat the underlying sepsis, and so is less important than antibiotics. A note about all questions in the exam; different departments have different antibiotic protocols, and this can be confusing. Unless there is a specific clue in the history, for example a history of listeria, therefore indicating amoxicillin as the best choice, you shouldn't get too hung up on the antibiotic being different from your local department policy, particularly if there is only one antibiotic choice. If you think sepsis is the diagnosis, you should treat it.

There are a large number of causes of anaemia in childhood. When you are faced with a question that asks you to identify the underlying cause of anaemia, you should approach this in a structured way. At the most basic level, anaemia is results from insufficient normally functioning red cells. This may be because insufficient numbers or quality of red cells are being produced, such as in nutritional deficiencies of iron or B12 and folate, or because of an underlying failure of production in the bone marrow, such as aplastic anaemia or red cell aplasia such as Diamond-Blackfan anaemia.

Alternatively, the red blood cells may be destroyed (haemolysed), in conditions such as haemolytic disease of the newborn, hereditary spherocytosis, or haemoglobinopathies such as sickle cell disease or the thalassaemias. In these conditions, knowledge of the epidemiology with respect to ethnicity is particularly important.

Finally, red blood cells may be removed through blood loss, which can be obvious, for example in trauma, or hidden, such as chronic low volume gastrointestinal blood loss. In neonates, twin-twin or feto-maternal transfusion can be causes of blood loss. An important cause of blood loss to consider in all children with frequent healthcare interactions is iatrogenic, and in girls, menstrual bleeding can result in anaemia.

Factors to consider when evaluating anaemia are dietary history, ethnicity, dysmorphic features, other underlying conditions (Inflammatory Bowel Disease for example), red cell indices, reticulocyte count, history of jaundice, and blood film appearances. Using this approach, you will be able to ascertain which broad group of aetiologies is likely, and then look for a condition from that group in the answer list.

Syllabus Mapping

Haematology and Oncology

- Know the causes and presentations of anaemia and their initial investigation and management

- Know how to interpret haematological investigations including full blood count, blood film and coagulation studies

Infection, Immunology and Allergy

- Know when antimicrobials are indicated

Neonatology

- Be able to recognise and initiate the management of common disorders in the newborn including sepsis

References and Further Reading

1. Essential Paediatric Haematology, Smith and Hann, 2002, Martin Dunitz Publishing

Chapter 50: Advice about feeding
Dr Heather Kitt and Dr James Blackburn

You are seeing patients in the primary care practice. Oliver is a 6 week old baby who is brought for his routine infant examination. He was born at term weighing 3.4 kg (25th - 50th Centile) with his weight now being 4.5 kg (25th centile). His routine examination is normal.

His mother is concerned about his weight gain. He wakes for a breast feeding every 3-4 hours and falls asleep after a feed. He has a good suck and feeds for 10-15 minutes. On reviewing his growth in his child health record, his only recorded weight was at 2 weeks of age when it was on the 25th centile.

Q1. Which one of the following is the most appropriate next step?

A.   Change to formula milk
B.   Start iron supplementation
C.   Vitamin D supplementation for Oliver
D.   Vitamin D supplementation for Oliver and his mother
E.   Vitamin D supplementation for Oliver's mother

Oliver remains well but aged 2 years you see him in the paediatric clinic following a referral by his GP.

"Please can you see Oliver who is sleeping a lot and is less active than usual when he is awake. His stools are variable between constipation and diarrhoea. He drinks 2 bottles of formula milk per day and eats a varied diet. He is not on any mediation nor supplements."

On examination his weight is 9.1 kg (0.4th centile). He has an erythematous rash with cracked skin at the angles of his mouth and has swollen wrists and he has developed a rash around his mouth. On examination, she also reports that his wrists appear more swollen.

Full blood count is as follows:

Haemoglobin	72 g/l
MCV	70 fl
Platelets	425 x 10⁹/l
Neutrophils	3.4 x 10⁹/l
Lymphocytes	4.5 x 10⁹/l

Q2. What nutritional deficiencies are likely based on Oliver's symptoms and signs?

A.   Calcium and Vitamin D
B.   Iron and Calcium
C.   Iron and Vitamin D
D.   Iron and Zinc
E.   Zinc and Vitamin D

Q3. What is the most likely cause of Oliver's symptoms?

A.   Autoimmune enteropathy
B.   Coeliac disease
C.   Dietary deficiency
D.   Inflammatory bowel disease
E.   Pancreatic insufficiency

Answers and Rationale

Q1. **D: Vitamin D supplementation for Oliver and his mother**
Q2. **C: Iron and Vitamin D**
Q3. **B: Coeliac disease**

Good infant nutrition is essential for growth and development and forms the foundation for long term health. Recent research suggests poor nutrition affects biological processes both in the short and long term, being associated with hypertension, obesity, insulin resistance, growth retardation, learning and cognition (1).

Breastfeeding is the gold standard for infant nutrition (WHO) and it is important to ensure mothers are aware of the benefits to both themselves and their child and are supported in breastfeeding for if possible. The benefits of breast feeding are well documented and include fewer childhood infections, increased intelligence, a probable protection against overweight and diabetes, and cancer prevention for mothers (2). It is estimated that the deaths of 823 000 children and 20 000 mothers deaths could be averted each year through universal breastfeeding, along with an economic savings of US$300 billion (2).

Current World Health recommendations are that infants should be exclusively breastfed for 6 months before introducing solids, with breastfeeding continuing until 2 years or beyond (3). The UK has one of the lowest rates of continuing breast feeding in the world with only 1 in 200 babies receiving any breast milk at the age of 12 months. By comparison, 27 per cent of babies in the USA, 35 per cent in Norway, 44 per cent in New Zealand and 92 per cent in India are breastfed until they are one year old (2).

Breastfed infants are at high risk of vitamin D deficiency as breast milk has low concentrations of vitamin D. Vitamin D is a fat-soluble vitamin that regulates calcium and phosphate homeostasis and is vital for musculoskeletal health. Children with insufficient exposure to sunlight and those with darker skin are at higher risk of vitamin D deficiency. Other risk factors include nutritional deficiency, certain comorbidities (e.g. malabsorption syndromes), and certain drugs (e.g. corticosteroids). Current UK advise is that all adults and children should take a daily supplement of vitamin D (4,5).

When you next see Oliver at 2 years of age he has developed faltering growth with features suggestive of malabsorption with nutritional deficiency. His full blood count demonstrates a microcytic anaemia, the commonest cause of which is iron deficiency. The rash in the corner of his mouth is describing angular chelitis, seen in both iron and zinc deficiency, though the relative frequency of both these conditions make iron deficiency the much more plausible answer. Thickening of the wrists, due to metaphyseal cartilage hyperplasia is one of the early signs of rickets. Other signs and symptoms include bone tenderness, muscle weakness, excessive bowing of the legs in toddlers and growth failure. Therefore Oliver has signs of both iron and Vitamin D deficiency resulting from malabsorption.

The most common cause of malabsorption is coeliac disease. The classical presentation is with loose stools and faltering growth which is progressive and may be seen when introducing new foods into the diet. There are however many potential presentations, which are often subtle as in Oliver's presentation. Symptoms include lethargy, irritability and depression. Coeliac disease is a multisystem disease and results in a small intestinal enteropathy due to gliadin exposure. This local inflammatory reaction produces flattened duodenal mucosa, loss of crypt architecture, glandular hyperplasia (crypts become deepened and elongated) and lymphocytosis of lamina propria in the proximal small bowel. This mucosal damage results in malabsorption of micronutrients (e.g., vitamins and minerals) and macronutrients (e.g. protein, carbohydrate, fat). Children with coeliac disease are at risk of deficiencies of vitamins such as zinc, folate and iron primarily absorbed in the jejunum as well as the fat-soluble vitamins A, D, E and K (6), for details about other these and other nutritional deficiencies (see table 50.1).

It is unlikely that Oliver has any of the other diagnoses in question 3. In autoimmune enteropathy, children usually experience severe vomiting and profuse diarrhoea. The normal lymphocyte and neutrophil count exclude this diagnosis (which would be reduced in autoimmune enteropathy). Pancreatic insufficiency in childhood is caused by a wide spectrum of pathologies, the most common being Cystic fibrosis, which would also have been likely detected by newborn screening). Given his symptomology it is unlikely that this is simple dietary deficiency and that there is an underlying medical diagnosis causing his nutrient deficiencies.

Nutrient	Dietary Source	Pathophysiology	Test Results	Clinical Presentation
Iron (7)	Red meat, dried fruit, fortified cereals, dried peas/beans Breast milk has ↓ concentration than formula but ↑ absorption.	Formation of; (i) haem molecule in haemoglobin and myoglobin; (ii) cytochromes for energy generation and drug metabolism. Absorbed mostly in the jejunum, and transported by transferrin. Stored in either ferritin or haemosiderin forms.	Microcytic hypochromic anaemia ↓ ferritin ↑ platelets	Anaemia, angular chelitis, weakness, poor growth, and generalised malaise. If severe anaemia bounding pulses, arrhythmia, and a systolic heart murmur and pica.
Folate (8)	Green leafy vegetables, orange juice, beans, legumes and liver.	Coenzyme, essential for DNA and RNA production.	Macrocytic anaemia	Anaemia, diarrhoea, peripheral neuropathy, mental confusion and depression. In pregnancy - neural tube defects, low birth weight, still birth and premature delivery.
Vitamin D (4,5)	Oily fish and eggs, margarine, fortified cereal, fortified formula and sunshine!	Cholecalciferol derived from diet and UV light conversion of 7 dehydrocholesterol, which is hydroxylated in the liver to 20-OH cholecalciferol and to 1,25 dihydroxycholecalciferol in the kidneys.	$\downarrow Ca^{2+}$ $\downarrow PO_4^{2-}$ Poor bone mineralisation with cupping and fraying	Rickets – growth stunting, tetany, muscle weakness, bone pain, increased fracture frequency. skeletal deformities (rachitic rosary, genu varum)

Nutrient	Dietary Source	Pathophysiology	Test Results	Clinical Presentation
Vitamin B12 (9)	Eggs, fish, meat, margarine	(i) aids in synthesis of methionine - important in neuronal function and formation of myelin (ii) conversion of methylmalonyl coenzyme A to succinyl coenzyme A (a key enzyme in the citric acid cycle – producing ATP).	Megaloblastic anaemia Howell-Jolly bodies, hypo plastic bone marrow pancytopenia. Pernicious anaemia.	Irritability, apathy, poor feeding, failure to thrive GI upset, developmental delay or regression + symptoms of pancytopenia (multiple infections, bleeding)
Zinc (10)	Nuts, seeds, lentils and fortified cereals Breast milk provides sufficient for the first 4-6 months of life but not after this	Action is not clearly understood, however is essential in catalytic, structural and regulatory functions, important in the function of enzymes and transcription factors. Also an anti-oxidant and may regulate the inflammatory process	↓ Zinc	Poor feeding, diarrhoea & abdominal pain, weight loss, osteopenia, increased infections, impaired wound-healing. Intention tremor. Depression, impaired concentration, nystagmus, dysarthria, night blindness, dementia. Pica.
Vitamin E (11)	Nuts, seeds and vegetable oils, green leafy vegetables and fortified cereals.	Essential in free radicle defence. Also enhances humoral and cell immune responses, phagocytic function and ↓ platelet aggregation.	↓ vitamin E Haemolytic anaemia in the preterm infant	Progressive neuropathy, hyporeflexia, muscle weakness and retinopathy. With severe deficiency, can get cardiac arrhythmias.
Vitamin K (12)	Bacteria in the GI tract. Dietary sources include green leafy vegetables	Synthesis of (i) clotting factors II,VII, IX, and X (ii) protein C and S, (anticoagulant). (iii) co-factor in the production of bone matrix proteins.	↑APPT ↑ PT ↓ prothrombin, factors VII, IX and X	Easy bruising, oozing from gums, nose or wounds - Haemorrhagic disease of the newborn.

Nutrient	Dietary Source	Pathophysiology	Test Results	Clinical Presentation
Vitamin A (13)	Liver, fish, eggs, milk products and yoghurt. Orange and yellow fruits/ and all green, leafy vegetables.	Provitamins A released from proteins in the stomach. Then hydrolysed to retinol in the small intestine. Retinaldehydes and retinoic acids required for normal vision, cell morphogenesis, growth, and differentiation.	↓ Retinol levels	Skin infections, throat infections, mouth ulcers, thrush, dandruff, dry hair, sore eyelids. Severe deficiency -- Night blindness, corneal opacification, bitot spots. growth failure, immune dysfunction.

Table 50.1: Information about Nutritional deficiencies

Syllabus Mapping

Nutrition

- Know the constituents of a healthy diet at all ages including breast and formula feeding in infancy

- Understand the principles of infant feeding

- Know the causes of malnutrition and understand the epidemiology and public health consequences of obesity

- Know the clinical presentation, and management of vitamin deficiencies

Gastroenterology and Hepatology

- Know the varied presentations of coeliac disease and its investigation and management

References and Further Reading

1. Fewtrell MS. The long-term benefits of having been breast-fed. Current paediatrics. 2004 Apr 30;14(2):97-103

2. Victora CG, Bahl R, Barros AJ, França GV, Horton S, Krasevec J, Murch S, Sankar MJ, Walker N, Rollins NC, Group TL. Breastfeeding in the 21st century: epidemiology, mechanisms, and lifelong effect. The Lancet. 2016 Feb 5;387(10017):475-90

3. GENEVA S. The optimal duration of exclusive breastfeeding. A systematic review. Geneva WHO. 2001

4. Vitamin D deficiency in adults - treatment and prevention. Nice clinical knowledge summary. November 2016

5. Vitamin D deficiency in children - treatment and prevention. Nice clinical knowledge summary. November 2016

6. Barker JM, Liu E. Celiac disease: pathophysiology, clinical manifestations and associated autoimmune conditions. Advances in pediatrics. 2008;55:349

7. Moy RJ, Early AR. Iron deficiency in childhood. Journal of the Royal Society of Medicine. 1999 May;92(5):234

8. Chan YM, Bailey R, O'Connor DL. Folate. Advances in Nutrition: An International Review Journal. 2013 Jan 1;4(1):123-5

9. Klee GG. Cobalamin and folate evaluation: measurement of methylmalonic acid and homocysteine vs vitamin B12 and folate. Clinical chemistry. 2000 Aug 1;46(8):1277-83

10. Roohani N, Hurrell R, Kelishadi R, Schulin R. Zinc and its importance for human health: An integrative review. Journal of Research in Medical Sciences. 2013 Feb 21;18(2):144-57

11. Rizvi S, ET AL., The Role of Vitamin E in Human Health and Some Diseases (2014) Sultan Qaboos Univ Med J.; 14(2): e157–e165. 12

12. Sutor AH, Von Kries R, Cornelissen EM, McNinch AW, Andrew M. Vitamin K deficiency bleeding (VKDB) in infancy. THROMBOSIS AND HAEMOSTASIS-STUTTGART-. 1999 Mar 1;81:456-61

13. Imdad A, Herzer K, Mayo-Wilson E, Yakoob MY, Bhutta ZA. Vitamin A supplementation for preventing morbidity and mortality in children from 6 months to 5 years of age. Cochrane Database Syst Rev. 2010 Jan 1;12

www.ingramcontent.com/pod-product-compliance
Lightning Source LLC
Chambersburg PA
CBHW082309210326

41599CB00029B/5743